Qigong
and Chinese
Self-Massage
for Everyday Health Care

of related interest

Principles of Chinese Medicine
What it is, how it works, and what it can do for you
Angela Hicks
ISBN 978 1 84819 130 3
eISBN 978 0 85701 107 7

Make Yourself Better
A Practical Guide to Restoring Your Body's
Wellbeing through Ancient Medicine
Philip Weeks
ISBN 978 1 84819 012 2
eISBN 978 0 85701 077 3

Qigong *and* Chinese Self-Massage

for Everyday Health Care

Ways to Address Chronic Health Issues
and to Improve Your Overall Health Based
on Chinese Medicine Techniques

Compiled by Zeng Qingnan

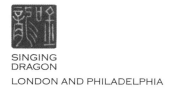

SINGING
DRAGON

LONDON AND PHILADELPHIA

This edition published in 2014
by Singing Dragon
an imprint of Jessica Kingsley Publishers
73 Collier Street
London N1 9BE, UK
and
400 Market Street, Suite 400
Philadelphia, PA 19106, USA

www.singingdragon.com

First published by Foreign Languages Press, Beijing, China, 1990

Library of Congress Cataloging in Publication Data
A CIP catalog record for this book is available from the Library of Congress

British Library Cataloguing in Publication Data
A CIP catalogue record for this book is available from the British Library

ISBN 978 1 84819 199 0

Printed and bound by Bell and Bain Ltd, Glasgow

Contents

Part Two: Methods of Keeping Fit

Foreword

Traditional Chinese medicine is by no means limited to herbal medication and acupuncture; its many branches of therapeutic methods include exercise therapies such as qigong and massage, which have an even longer history than medication. They were not only recorded in medical literature but have also been handed down and widely disseminated among the Chinese as self-health care measures because of their simplicity and effectiveness. In this book, the editor has selected only a limited number of these exercises.

Most of the diseases that can be prevented and treated by these measures are "minor" problems, not so serious as cancers and cardiovascular seizures. However, these "minor" problems are so common that they cause great suffering and enormous economic loss if the whole community is considered. "Health for all by the year 2000," advocated by the World Health Organization (WHO), became the common goal of people all over the world. One of the fundamental approaches to meeting this goal was the participation of people at the community level; they need to have easy access to simple methods that will improve their health. This collection of health care measures can partly meet this requirement.

Whether they are culled from classical literature or derived from folk remedies, all the health care methods in this book are described within the framework of traditional Chinese medical theories, particularly the theory of meridians and collaterals and the theory of qi. Qi has different implications in different contexts. In most instances, qi refers to the vital energy of the human body, which serves as the motive element or force behind life activities and internal functions. Qigong also has many varieties. In this book, qigong is an exercise that mobilizes and directs the flow of qi through concentration of the mind and regulation of respiration for preventive and therapeutic purposes.

Meridians and collaterals are the conduit system for the circulation of qi and blood. Along the meridians there are certain points that the qi of the internal organs can reach. Because acupuncturists use these points, they are called acupoints. Although no acupuncture is involved in this book, there are many instructions for digital pressing, kneading, massaging and performing other manipulations of the acupoints. I have adopted in my translation the Standard Acupuncture Nomenclature recommended by WHO Working Groups and published by the WHO Regional Office for the Western Pacific. The standard nomenclature of acupoints consists of the Chinese phonetic (Pinyin) name, followed by the alphanumeric code in parenthesis, but the Chinese characters have been omitted. The English language names of the 14 meridians and their alphabetic codes are as follows:

Lung Meridian L	Large Intestine Meridian LI
Stomach Meridian S	Spleen Meridian Sp
Heart Meridian H	Small Intestine Meridian SI
Bladder Meridian B	Kidney Meridian K
Pericardium Meridian P	Triple Energizer Meridian TE
Gallbladder Meridian G	Liver Meridian Liv
Governor Vessel GV	Conception Vessel CV

If readers are interested in more detail about the acupoints, monographs on acupuncture can be consulted using either the Chinese phonetic names or alphanumeric codes for reference.

Some (but not all) of the extra points—that is, acupoints later identified and nominated other than those of the 14 main meridians—have alphanumeric codes initiated by "Ex" according to the Standard Acupuncture Nomenclature.

Because location of the acupoints is so important, that information is noted for each one mentioned in this book, using cun as the unit of measurement. In traditional Chinese medicine, there are two ways of defining cun. In the first way, one cun is equivalent to the distance between the joint creases of the interphalangeal joints of the patient's middle finger when it is flexed, as used in the following descriptions:

"Yingxiang (LI 20) is located in the nasolabial fold, 0.5 cun lateral to the ala nasi"; "Taiyang (Ex-HN 5) is in the depression one cun lateral to the external canthus of the eye (HN is the abbreviation for 'head and neck')." In the other method, one cun equals the length of a division of the patient's body when the body is divided into sections of equal length. For example, from the umbilicus to the upper border of the symphysis pubis equals five cun; thus the statement "Qihai (CV 6) is 1.5 cun below the umbilicus" means that Qihai (CV 6) is at the upper three-tenths of the line joining the umbilicus and the upper border of the symphysis pubis.

Though somewhat technical in nature, the information included here will be, I believe, of immediate and practical use. It is my sincere wish that the positive effects of these methods in preventing and treating a series of common diseases will be felt by many more people with the translation and publication of this material in English.

Professor Xie Zhufan

Part One

Methods of
Curing Diseases

1

Treatment of Gray Hair

There is a saying in traditional Chinese medicine that hair is the odds and ends of blood. In other words, hair is nourished by blood.

In the Qin Dynasty, Zhang Zihe (1156–1228) in his *Ru Men Shi Qing* (Confucians' Duties to Their Parents) said: "If a young man is gray-headed, has lost his hair or has a lot of dandruff, there is excess heat in the blood." In the Ming Dynasty, Li Chan in *Yi Xue Ru Men* (Elementary Medicine) (1575) explained further: "Exuberant blood flow nourishes the hair, making it moist and lustrous, whereas an insufficient blood supply withers it. Heat in the blood causes the hair to become yellowish, and further derangement of the blood gives rise to whitening of the hair."

Since having gray hair is closely related to insufficient blood flow, the goal of the treatment should be to restore the hair to its original color. Traditional literature suggests that Daoyin (physical and breathing exercise), which promotes the circulation of qi and blood, is beneficial for this condition. The following methods are recommended.

Method I

Method I, described in Zhou Lujing's *Xiao Yao Zi Dao Yin Jue* (Formula for Physical and Breathing Exercise), was written in the early seventeenth century.

Perform the exercise twice a day, at 1 a.m. and 12 noon. Sit upright with the hands holding each other (see Fig. 1). Concentrate and empty your mind of all distractions. In your mind's eye, look at your own vertex and you will feel naturally the qi of Yin and Yang running along the spine from the sacrum up to the vertex, down to the ridge of the nose, chin and throat, and along the anterior midline of the chest and abdomen to Dantian—3 cun below the umbilicus. After nine circulations of qi, you will be full of vigor. Consistent practice may restore gray hair to its original color.

Method II

Method II, recorded in *Zhu Bing Yuan Hou Lun* (General Treatise on the Causes and Symptoms of Diseases) (610), has three different exercises.

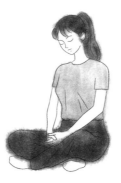 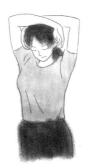

Fig. 1   Fig. 2

1. After getting up in the morning, raise the right arm and bend it over the head to hold the left ear; at the same time, raise the

left arm and bend it over the head to hold the right ear. Lift both ears simultaneously. Then pull the hair (see Fig. 2). This exercise can promote qi and blood circulation in the hair.

2. Sit on the ground with the legs and arms stretched straight ahead and the fingers pointing to the feet. Bend over and try to touch the head to the ground, thus exercising the spine to prevent disease and improving qi and blood circulation in the hair follicles to promote hair growth. Then, sit on a chair with the legs relaxed and the feet spaced 30 cm apart, and hold the lower legs just above the ankles with the hands. Bend over with the head pointing towards the ground (see Fig. 3). Repeat 12 times. This movement of the spine is beneficial for preventing disease and allowing essential qi to nourish the hair so that it remains shiny and soft.

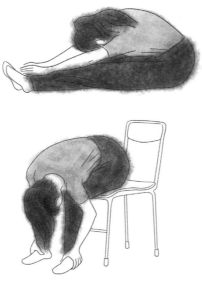

Fig. 3

3. Bend the knees to form a right angle as if sitting, but do not let the buttocks touch the ground. Bend over, hold the toes and turn them up with the hands. Then bend the head down towards the ground as far as possible (see Fig. 4). This practice can direct the qi of all the internal organs to the head and is helpful for the treatment of deafness and blurred vision. Consistent practice will also restore gray hair to its original color.

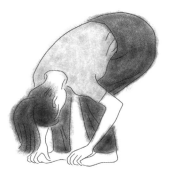

Fig. 4

Method III

Method III, from *Yan Shou Shu* (On Prolonging the Life), is frequent combing of the hair.

Combing the hair promotes metabolism of the scalp and the hair roots (see Fig. 5). In reality, however, massage of the scalp is more effective. Before going to bed in the evening and after getting up in the morning, use the index and middle fingers to apply circular massage on the scalp, from the forehead through the vertex to the occipital region, and then from the forehead through bilateral Taiyang (Ex-HN 5) (in the depression 1 cun lateral to the external canthus of the eye) to the occipital region (see Fig. 6). Perform the practice twice a day, 10 to 15 minutes each time, and 30 to 40 turns of massage each minute. Long-term and consistent practice will achieve good effects. Scalp massage improves blood circulation, supplies the hair papillae with additional nutrients, increases the production of melanin and facilitates its transport, thus restoring gray hair to its original color.

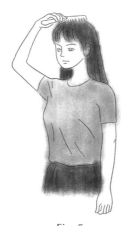

Fig. 5

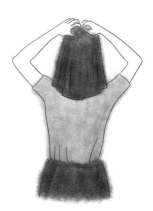

Fig. 6

2

Treatment of Myopia
with Still Qigong

How can myopia be treated with still qigong? Traditional Chinese medical theory states that all human biological activities depend on blood circulation and qi promotion. Blood will not flow if qi is obstructed. Still qigong mobilizes and concentrates the essential qi of the internal organs in the human body, promotes its flow in the channels and collaterals, and regulates qi and blood to normalize blood circulation and supply the eyes with adequate nutrients. Thus, the tension of the eyes will be relieved and accommodation restored.

The essentials for treating myopia with still qigong are as follows: to practice relaxation, still qigong first relaxes the body and makes the mind tranquil to normalize the qi and blood; then it guides the qi to the hands, and finally regulates the qi and blood of the ocular muscles by emitting external qi through the hands. Once qigong is properly practiced, the "feeling of qi" will soon be experienced.

Still qigong is characterized by its simplicity, safety and beneficial effects on true myopia, pseudomyopia and hereditary myopia in both young people and adults.

The qigong treatment of myopia consists of three steps: practice of qi cultivation in still standing; practice of qi guidance by opening and closing; and practice of eye massage with external qi.

I. Practice of qi cultivation in still standing

Stand erect with the legs together and the feet slightly turned out. The big toes should be spaced about a fist's width apart. Relax the knees and put the feet flat and the body weight on the bilateral sole centers.

Tuck the hips in and don't let the hip joints turn forwards.

Draw the buttocks in and don't let them protrude backwards.

Keep the spine straight, the waist and abdomen relaxed and the chest extended.

Keep the head upright, the neck straight, the chin tucked in, the ears in line with the shoulders, the tip of the nose pointing to the umbilicus, the eyes and mouth gently shut, the tongue touching the palate, and breathe naturally.

Don't square the shoulders. Drop the arms naturally and place one little finger by each side seam of the trousers, with the back of the hand slanting to the anterior, all the fingers relaxed, the center of the palm hollowed, and the middle finger extending naturally. Keep the arms extended and relaxed (see Fig. 1).

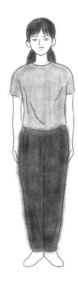

Fig. 1

The key points of this practice are to keep the head upright, body straight, feet flat and arms extended so that the upper and lower parts of the body are linked in physical relaxation and the mind is concentrated on relaxing naturally. Practice for about 15 minutes each time.

II. Practice of qi guidance by opening and closing

Stand still with the tips of the toes together; then raise the left foot, move it to the left, and put it down so that the feet are parallel and about shoulder width apart.

Gradually raise the hands forwards and upwards until they reach shoulder level (see Fig. 2).

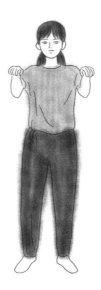

Fig. 2

Bend the knees slightly, sinking down to a sitting position, and at the same time relax the shoulders, drop the elbows and make the arms semicircular. Keep the wrists level with the shoulders, palms facing each other. Note the opposition and union of Laogong (P 8) between the two palms (see Fig. 3).

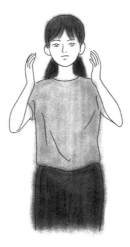

Fig. 3

Relax the hands until some feeling of numbness, distension or hotness appears. Then slowly bring the hands together as if pressing on a balloon until the distance between the palm centers is shortened to 6 or 7 cm (action of closing). Next, slowly move the hands apart to shoulder width (action of opening). Then "close" the palms again. Repeat opening and closing in this way for about 5 minutes. A feeling of difficulty in moving the hands or in the actions of opening and closing will be experienced (see Figs 4 and 5).

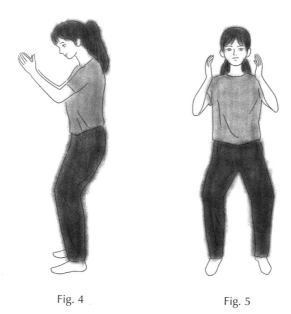

Fig. 4   Fig. 5

The practice of qi guidance aims to make the inner and outer qi work in consonance, so that not only can the internal organs be reinforced by regulating the flow of qi in the channels, but myopia can also be treated by the outer qi being guided by will.

III. Practice of eye massage with external qi

Take off your spectacles. This therapy can be divided into five sections.

1. When there is a strong feeling of qi in the palms, slowly turn the hands over, directing Laogong (P 8) to the eyes. Holding the qi in the palms, slowly move the hands close to the eyes until the palms are 6 to 12 cm away from the eyes and there is a feeling of pressure or hotness in the eyes. Practice for one minute to cause the qi to go from the palms deep into the eyeballs and to combine with the qi already inside the eyes (see Fig. 6).

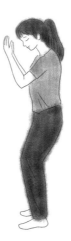

Fig. 6

2. Having felt the combination of the qi in the palms and in the eyeballs, slowly move the hands away until they are about 40 cm from the eyes, to pull the qi out; then slowly press the qi into the eyeballs until the palms are about 6 cm away from the eyes. Slowly pull and press in this manner six to nine times (see Fig. 7), finally stopping at a distance about 15 cm away from the eyes. During pulling and pressing, there is a feeling of attraction and resistance that is different in strength in different people (see Fig. 8).

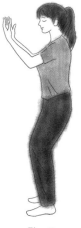
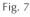
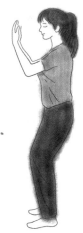

Fig. 7

Fig. 8

3. Keep the distance between the hands and the eyes unchanged. Feeling the union of qi between the hands and eyes, slowly turn both hands in the same direction in a circular movement first to the left and then to the right, three to six times each. The radius of the circular movement should be short enough so that the qi in the palms can drive the qi in the eyes, giving rise to a feeling of rotation (see Fig. 9).

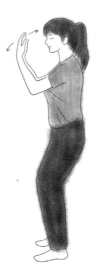

Fig. 9

4. Stop the circular movement and keep the palms still at the same distance, facing the eyes. Relax the whole body and become aware as the qi of the palms is transported to the eyes and deeply into the eyeballs, which results in regulation of qi and blood and improvement of the functions of the eye. Practice the eye massage with external qi for about 5 minutes (see Fig. 10).

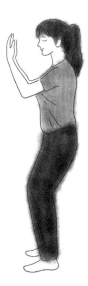

Fig. 10

5. To close the movement, slowly raise the palms and keep them close to the eyes for one minute. Rub the eyes with both palms in the same direction, first to the left three times and then to the right three times (see Fig. 11). After a short pause, move the hands downwards with the middle fingers passing Jingming (B 1) in the depression 0.1 cun medial to the inner canthi, along the sides of the nose to the chest and abdomen (see Fig. 12).

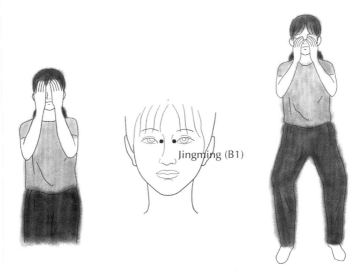

Jingming (B1)

Fig. 11   Fig. 12

Place the legs together, separate the hands and turn the feet out slightly, restoring the original posture of standing still. After a little while, slowly open the eyes, looking to the left, to the right and to the front. Your vision will be clear and bright.

This whole set of exercises takes about 30 minutes. Practice twice a day, in the morning and in the evening.

Still qigong can be performed at any time, before or after meals, in the morning or evening, or during a break at work or between classes. If it is done as an exercise between classes, stand still for 2 or 3 minutes, and then make the inner and outer qi work in consonance by qi guidance and massage the eyes with the outer qi. Practice 5 to 10 minutes each time. It is better for beginners to practice qi guidance more, at least 5 minutes each time, until the feeling of qi has become very strong immediately after "closing" the palms. Then they should practice eye massage more than qi guidance. Consistent practice for more than three months usually gives a stable therapeutic effect. However, prevention of eyestrain is also important. Neglecting eye hygiene will cause a recurrence of myopia.

3

A Therapeutic Exercise
for a Stiff Neck

Many people suffer with a stiff neck: sharp pains and a feeling of distension in the neck, greatly aggravated by turning the head, and sometimes accompanied by a stretching pain radiating to the back and shoulder. In serious cases, the head is immovable and can be turned only together with the trunk.

Stiff neck often occurs in the following conditions:

1. Sleeping on a high pillow with overfatigue, keeping some muscles of the neck and back (mainly the sternocleidomastoid and trapezius muscles) in a position of overextension for a long time and stagnation of qi and blood caused by an attack of wind-cold.

2. Long periods of reading or working with the head falling forward, leading to chronic strain of the neck muscles.

3. Sudden turning of the head causing a sprain of the neck muscles.

Generally speaking, once a stiff neck occurs, its frequent recurrence is common if no effective preventive measures are taken. Furthermore, a patient with cervical spondylitis usually has a recurrent stiff neck.

Many people do not consider a stiff neck a disease and usually seek treatment only after several days' delay. In fact, application of exercise therapy immediately after the onset of the stiff neck will give a prompt, satisfactory effect.

Instructions

Step I: Don't be afraid of pain. Slowly move the head in the direction of the stiffness to stretch the affected muscles. Turn the head and massage yourself, first pressing and kneading the tender point with the thumb and then kneading all the involved muscles with the palm. Meanwhile, bend the head forwards or backwards wherever there is pain.

Step II: After improving the cervical movement, perform the following therapeutic exercises:

1. CLENCHING FISTS AND BENDING ELBOWS

Preparatory posture: Stand naturally with the arms hanging down.

Movements: (1) Clench fists and at the same time bend the elbows; extend the arms backwards with force (see Fig. 1). (2) Resume the preparatory posture.

2. Tilting the Head Forwards and Backwards

Preparatory posture: Stand naturally with arms akimbo.

Movements: (1) After bending the head forwards, slowly lift it up and tilt it backwards with force (see Fig. 2). (2) Resume the preparatory posture.

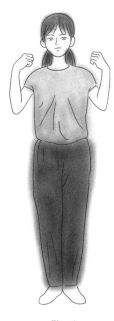
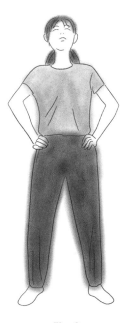

Fig. 1   Fig. 2

3. STRIKING DIAGONALLY WITH FISTS

Preparatory posture: Stand with the feet apart, clench fists and bend the elbows in a right angle.

Movements: (1) Turn the body to the right, striking to the right and forwards with the left fist, and then resume the preparatory posture. (2) Turn the body to the left, striking to the left and forwards with the right fist, and then return to the preparatory posture (see Fig. 3).

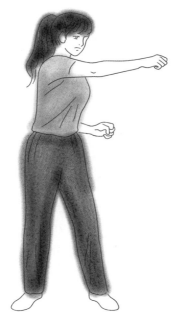

Fig. 3

4. Turning the head to the left and to the right

Preparatory posture: Stand with arms akimbo and feet apart.

Movements: (1) Turn the head to the left and then resume the original position. (2) Turn the head to the right and then resume the original position (see Fig. 4).

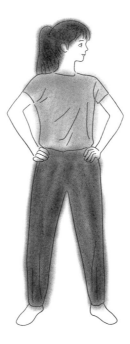

Fig. 4

5. "SUPPORTING THE SKY WITH PALMS"

Preparatory posture: Stand with the arms hanging down naturally and the feet apart.

Movements: (1) Place the hands in front of the abdomen with the palms facing up and the fingers of the left and right hands pointing towards each other. Slowly raise the hands to chest level and turn the hands with the palms facing up again while extending the arms until the elbows become straight (see Fig. 5). (2) Resume the preparatory posture.

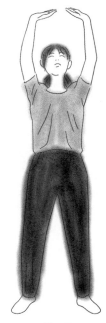

Fig. 5

6. "LOOKING AT THE MOON WITH THE HEAD TURNED AROUND"

Preparatory posture: Stand with the arms hanging down naturally and the feet apart.

Movements: (1) Tilt the body forwards with the knees slightly bent. Turn the upper torso to the left and support the back of the head with the right hand. Then turn the head with the eyes looking upwards and backwards. (2) Reverse the actions, turning to the right (see Fig. 6).

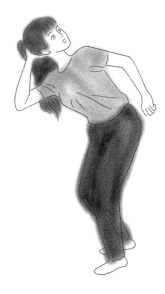

Fig. 6

7. LIFTING THE SHOULDERS AND ROTATING THEM BACKWARDS

Preparatory posture: Stand with the arms hanging down naturally and the feet apart.

Movements: (1) Lift the shoulders and rotate them backwards. (2) Relax the shoulders and resume the preparatory posture (see Fig. 7).

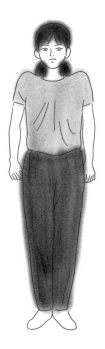

Fig. 7

8. "Shooting with a bow"

Preparatory posture: Stand with the arms hanging down naturally and the feet apart.

Movements: (1) Bend the knees and turn the upper torso to the left. Meanwhile, raise the forearms in front of the body with the left hand on top and the right hand below, palms facing each other. When the forearms reach chest level, pull the right hand down and backwards and push the left hand up and to the left, as if shooting with a bow, with the eyes looking at the left hand. (2) Resume the preparatory posture. Reverse the actions, turning to the right (see Fig. 8).

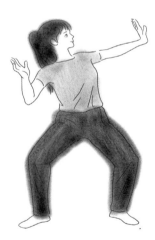

Fig. 8

9. RAISING THE ARM AND KNEE

Preparatory posture: Stand with the arms hanging down naturally and the feet apart.

Movements: (1) Raise the right arm sideways above the head and turn the hand over, the palm facing upward. Meanwhile, raise the left knee. (2) Resume the original posture. Then raise the left arm and the right knee (see Fig. 9).

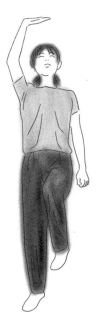

Fig. 9

10. RESISTING AGAINST THE NAPE

Preparatory posture: Stand with the feet apart and place the hands behind the head at the nape with the fingers interlocked.

Movements: (1) Slowly bend the head backwards with force, resisting against the head with the hands. (2) Resume the original posture and then repeat the exercise (see Fig. 10).

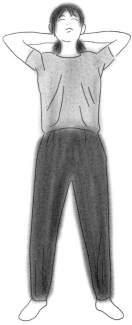

Fig. 10

Perform the exercise set once a day, repeating each action 12 to 16 times. The actions should be practiced slowly, producing a stretching feeling in the muscles of the neck.

The goals of these therapeutic exercises are to stretch the neck muscles and remove spasm, to balance bilateral muscular tone, to restore the physiological curvature of the cervical vertebrae, to relieve pain and to restore the functional activities of the neck and shoulders.

4

Prevention and Treatment of Cervical Spondylosis by Writing a Chinese Character

Cervical spondylosis is a common disease in middle-aged and older people. It is often caused by overfatigue or exposure to wind-cold or injury and is characterized by nervous and vasomotor disturbances manifested as soreness and numbness of the head, neck, shoulders, arms and hands in mild cases, and muscular atrophy or even paralysis of the upper extremities in severe cases, leading to disability.

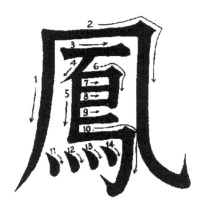

All cervical spondylosis patients suffer from the inability to freely turn the head, which interferes with their daily life and work.

In Western medicine, the common treatment is to reduce the pressure by traction. In traditional Chinese medicine, massage therapy is used together with movement with the doctor's assistance. These treatment techniques are certainly effective, but the patients have to visit the clinic frequently.

Since ancient times, an effective self-treatment of cervical spondylosis has been handed down as a folk remedy in China.

I. Preliminary exercise

1. Rubbing the shoulders: Rub the shoulders with the fingers 30 times. Rub the left shoulder with the right hand and the right shoulder with the left hand (see Fig. 1).

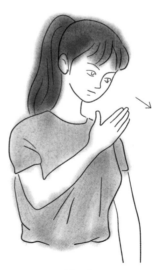

Fig. 1

2. Pinching and lifting Jianjing (G 21): Pinch and lift this point several times. Jianjing (G 21) is in the depression of the trapezius, superior to the superior angle of the scapula (see Fig. 2).

3. Looking to the left and to the right: Turn the head to the left with the eyes looking to the rear and up, and then turn to the right with the eyes looking to the rear and up. The actions should be slow and the extent of the movement as large as possible (see Fig. 3).

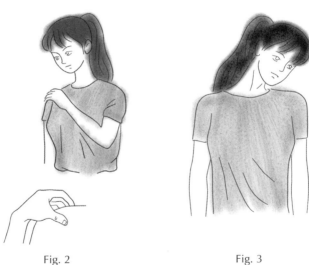

Fig. 2   Fig. 3

4. Backward extension: Bend the head slightly forward, and then slowly extend it backwards as far as possible. After a forceful contraction of the nuchal muscles, restore the head to its original position. Repeat the action 20 times (see Fig. 4).

5. Turning the neck slowly: Perform this action slowly and increase the extent of the movement gradually. Repeat the action for 5 to 10 minutes (see Fig. 5).

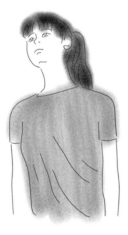
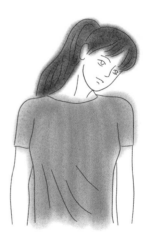

Fig. 4   Fig. 5

This preliminary exercise of the neck and nape is easy to do. It can achieve the same result as traction therapy in Western medicine, increasing the strength of the cervical muscles and the stability of the neck.

II. Writing a Chinese character with the head

After finishing the preliminary exercise, perform the following movements:

Taking the cervical vertebrae as the axis and fully relaxing the head, swing the neck in a large arc to make the head and neck move upwards and downwards to the left and to the right as far as possible.

Then move the head and neck in the following order:

1. Move the head in a downward direction, as if writing a down stroke of 丿.

2. Move the head horizontally from the left to the right and then from top to bottom as if writing the stroke 乚.

3. Move the head as if to write strokes 一 , 丿 , 丨 , and ㇇.

4. Move the head to write three horizontal strokes 三, followed by 乛, and finally four dots from left to right 灬. Thus, the Chinese character 鳳 is written.

The Chinese character 鳳 means phoenix, a mythical bird with extremely beautiful feathers, considered to be the king of birds and an auspicious sign. This character is chosen because of its complex strokes in various directions, which give sufficient exercise to the cervical vertebrae.

Perform the exercise two or three times a day, writing the character 鳳 with the head three times at each session. Consistent practice will achieve good results.

5

Exercise for Periarthritis of the Shoulder

After reaching the age of 45 one often feels pain in the shoulders, has difficulty moving the joints and is sometimes unable to raise the shoulders or experiences limitation when attempting to extend the arms upwards. This is called periarthritis of the shoulder, a common condition in middle-aged people. Since it often occurs from about the age of 45, and especially after the age of 50, it is known in China as the "50-year-old shoulder." It is also known as "frozen shoulder."

In traditional Chinese medicine, the effect of wind-cold on the shoulder is thought to be the major cause of this condition.

A person above the age of 45 usually does less physical activity and exercise, especially if suffering from a chronic condition. Decreased movement of the shoulders and arms impairs the local blood circulation and supply of nutrients, resulting in chronic degenerative changes of the shoulder joint and its surrounding soft tissues. Meanwhile, a middle-aged person also begins to have a lower rate of metabolism and the general condition of the body begins to decline, including the shoulder joint. Once the shoulder is attacked by wind-cold, periarthritis occurs.

The patient usually feels local pain in the shoulder involved, accompanied by a sensation of heaviness. The pain is aggravated at night, impairing sleep. During the day, raising or outward turning of the arm causes sharp pain, affecting not only work but also daily life.

There is no special drug therapy for this condition at present. The following exercise can be helpful for the recovery of the shoulder's functions. The patient may perform the total series or just sections of the exercise.

1. Swing the arms: Stand with the feet shoulder width apart and gently swing the arms back and forth with a gradual increase in the size of the swing. Perform twice a day, in the morning and in the evening, 50 to 100 swings each time (see Fig. 1).

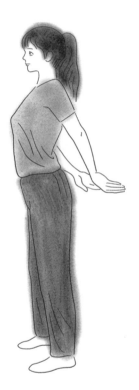

Fig. 1

2. Picking up things: Stand with the feet shoulder width apart and bend the upper torso forwards. Move the affected forearm(s) downwards as if picking up something. Perform twice a day, in the morning and in the evening, 30 to 50 actions each time (see Fig. 2).

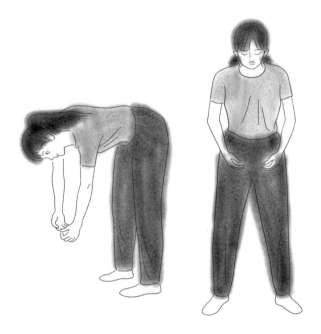

Fig. 2

3. Drawing circles: Stand with the feet shoulder width apart and keep the torso still. Move the arms forwards and backwards as if drawing circles, gradually increasing the size of the circles. Perform twice a day, drawing 50 to 100 circles each time (see Fig. 3).

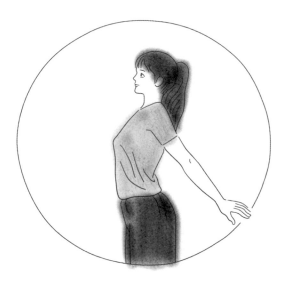

Fig. 3

4. Touching the wall: Stand by the wall and touch it with the affected hand from the bottom to the top, reaching as high as possible. Repeat 20 to 30 times (see Fig. 4).

5. Shrugging the shoulders: Sit or stand. Bend the elbows in a 90-degree angle and then shrug the shoulders with increasing force. Perform twice a day, 50 to 100 shrugs each time (see Fig. 5).

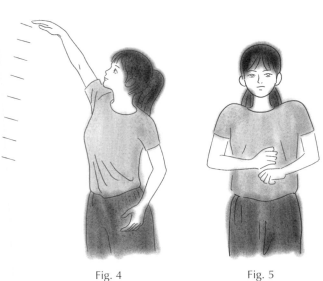

Fig. 4   Fig. 5

6. Touching the height: Hang something on a tree or in the room. Raise the affected arm as far as possible to touch it, gradually increasing the height. Practice twice a day, 50 to 100 touches each time (see Fig. 6).

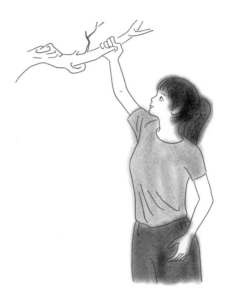

Fig. 6

7. "Upward-shooting gun": Sit or stand with the hands holding each other. Place the hands above the head and then gradually stretch the arms straight, extending the hands over the head as far as possible. Repeat 30 to 50 times (see Fig. 7).

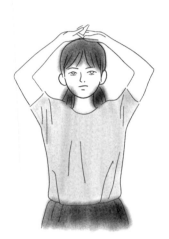 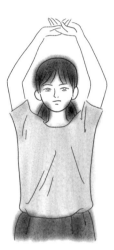

Fig. 7

8. "Spreading the wings": Stand with the feet shoulder width apart. Straighten the arms and raise them to the sides to form an angle of 90 degrees between the arm and the torso. Lower the arms after 5 to 10 seconds. Repeat 30 to 50 times a day (see Fig. 8).

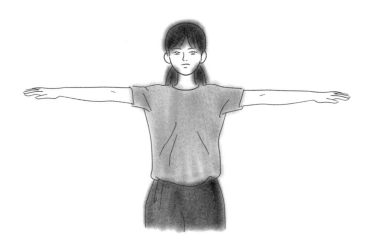

Fig. 8

9. Touching the nape: Sit or stand. Touch the nape with the left and right hands alternately. Practice twice a day, 50 to 100 touches each time (see Fig. 9).

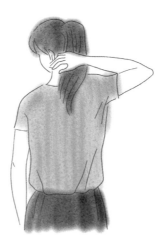

Fig. 9

6

Patting to Treat Shoulder Pain and Backache

Pain in the shoulder and lower back in functional disorders, with the exception of that caused by organic lesions, is usually caused by muscle spasm, nonbacterial inflammation and tissue contracture. According to traditional Chinese medicine, these pains are caused by qi stagnation and blood stasis in the meridians and collaterals, which result from the invasion of wind-cold into the shoulders and back.

Sun Simiao, the most famous physician in the Tang Dynasty, wrote in his *Qianjin Yao Fang* (One Thousand Golden Prescriptions): "For one with a feeling of coldness in the hands, pat them hot from top to bottom"; "For one feeling coldness in the feet, also pat them hot." That is to say, massage by patting can be used in the treatment of these conditions.

"Heat promotes blood flow" and "Cold syndromes should be treated with heat" are general principles in traditional treatment. In other words, blood circulation needs warmth, and the diseases caused by cold should be treated by warmth.

The following four steps of patting, designed in accordance with this theory, are effective for the treatment of pain in the shoulders and lower back.

Instructions

1. Patting the arms: Stand naturally with the feet apart. Raise one arm horizontally, but do not stretch it straight. Pat it with the other palm from the shoulder to the wrist and hand, and then back from the hand to the shoulder along the anterior, lateral and posterior aspects. Use alternate patting on the left and right arms, and repeat 12 to 24 times (see Fig. 1).

This exercise promotes the circulation of qi and blood in the shoulders and arms, releases adhesions and hence reduces soreness and pain.

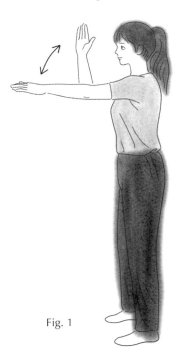

Fig. 1

2. Pounding the shoulders and back: Stand naturally with the feet apart. Pat on the left shoulder with the right palm, at the same time giving light blows on the right side of the back with the back of the left hand. Alternate patting on the left and right sides and repeat 12 to 24 times (see Fig. 2).

This exercise relaxes the shoulders and back, relieves spasms, soothes the tendons and therefore alleviates soreness and pain.

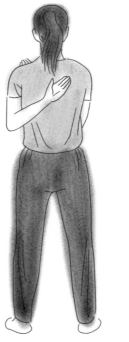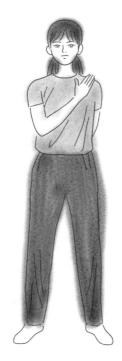

Fig. 2

3. Knocking on Shenshu (B 23): Stand naturally with the feet apart. Knock on the left and right Shenshu (B 23) (on the lower back, 1.5 cun lateral to the midpoint between the spinous processes of the second and third lumbar vertebrae) alternately with the palms, the back of the hand or the back of the fist (see Fig. 3). Repeat 12 to 24 times.

This exercise strengthens the kidneys, promotes blood circulation, relieves numbness and is therefore good for the treatment of lower back pain.

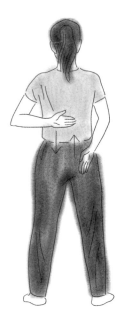

Fig. 3

4. Swaying the waist while swinging the arms: Stand naturally with the feet apart and relax the whole body. Swing the arms to the left and to the right alternately while swaying the waist. Beat the waist with the swinging hands, particularly delivering blows on the lower back with the back of the hands (see Fig. 4). Repeat 12 to 24 times.

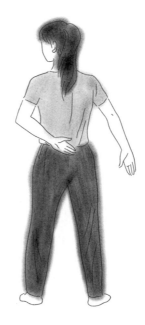

Fig. 4

This exercise is designed to relax the sacrum and hips, soothe the tendons, strengthen the waist, prevent disease and ensure longevity.

The duration and frequency of this exercise will be different for different people. It is enough when a feeling of hotness occurs. Generally speaking, each exercise session takes about 20 minutes, and the exercise should be done two to four times a day, half an hour before or after meals.

Notes

1. Patting and pounding should be done slowly without tension, moving gradually from light to heavy blows.

2. The exercise load can be adjusted in the following way: Add more if there is only soreness, reduce if there is pain and stop if there is numbness. When there is muscle soreness with a feeling of heaviness and distension while raising the arms (this is a normal reaction to the exercise), the exercise load should be increased. Increased local pain indicates an incipient inflammation of muscles or tendons, and the exercise load should be reduced to avoid extension of the inflammation. Numbness is a sign of pressure on a local nerve, suggesting incorrect practice. Stop the exercise at once to find out the cause and resume practicing only when the faults have been corrected.

3. Be sure to take off your top layers of clothing before exercising. In the winter, you may leave a top layer on until after one or two steps and put it back on immediately after exercising to avoid catching cold. Change your undershirt if it has been dampened by sweat.

Contraindications

1. Stop exercising if there is acute local inflammation, high temperature or symptoms of hemorrhage.

2. Do not perform these exercises during times of emotional upset; the requirements of the movements cannot properly be achieved, and excessive actions may cause injury.

This kind of patting is especially suitable for older people with weak constitutions and soreness in the back, shoulders and arms. Though simple, it offers good results if it is performed consistently.

7

Abdomen-Kneading
A Remedy for Gastrointestinal Diseases

Abdomen-kneading is a form of health-protecting manipulation that has been popular in China since the seventeenth century.

This practice is chiefly aimed at massaging the internal organs, promoting blood circulation in the abdomen and stimulating the gastrointestinal and mesenteric neuroreceptors by kneading and pressing acupoints and areas of the abdomen. Stimulation of the neuroreceptors can induce vagus excitation, which promotes contraction of the smooth muscles of the gastrointestinal tract and its peristalsis; increases gastric, biliary, pancreatic and small-intestinal secretions; enhances digestion and absorption; and elevates carbohydrate, protein and fat metabolism and detoxication in the liver.

The practice of abdomen-kneading is effective for treating peptic ulcer, chronic gastritis, gastric neurosis, colitis, habitual constipation and other gastrointestinal diseases.

I. Posture during practice

Sit or lie supine. In a sitting position, keep the upper part of the body upright and place the feet flat on the ground, spaced at a little more than shoulder width apart. In a supine position, slightly bend the knees and keep the feet apart with the heels touching the bed. In cold weather, it is better to be supine, covered with a quilt while kneading the abdomen.

II. Manipulations

1. Kneading Zhongwan (CV 12): Place the palmar aspect of the right index, middle and ring fingertips on the epigastrium, and on these fingers place the left index, middle and ring fingers. Press with both hands and gently knead around Zhongwan (CV 12), making 36 circles clockwise. (Zhongwan is located at the midpoint between the upper border of the xyphoid process and the umbilicus; see Figs 1 and 2.)

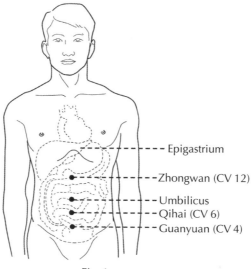

Epigastrium

Zhongwan (CV 12)

Umbilicus
Qihai (CV 6)
Guanyuan (CV 4)

Fig. 1

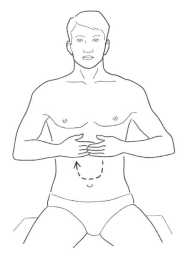

Fig. 2

2. Kneading the umbilicus: Using the right index, middle and ring fingertips, gently knead around the umbilicus in circular movements clockwise, starting from the left side of the umbilicus and drawing 18 circles. Also press the right-hand fingers with the three corresponding fingers of the left hand while kneading. Then knead with the left hand, starting from the right side of the umbilicus and kneading counterclockwise for 18 circles.

3. Kneading Qihai (CV 6) and Guanyuan (CV 4): Knead with the right index, middle and ring fingers (while pressing these fingers with the corresponding fingers of the left hand), starting from Qihai (CV 6), 1.5 cun below the umbilicus, moving to the left and downwards, passing through Guanyuan (CV 4),

3 cun below the umbilicus, and then moving to the right and upwards, back to Qihai (CV 6), forming a circle. After 18 circular movements, gently knead with the left hand counterclockwise for another 18 circles.

4. Pushing Conception Vessel Renmai: Using the index, middle and ring fingers of one hand while pressing these fingers with the corresponding fingers of the other hand, gently push from the epigastrium along the anterior midline down to the symphysis pubis. Part the hands and move outwards along the bilateral iliac fossae while kneading with the index, middle and ring fingers. Then move upwards along the inframammary lines to the costal arches while kneading with rotatory movements. One cycle is completed when the hands come back to the epigastrium and resume their original position—that is, the index, middle and ring fingers of one hand are pressed on the corresponding fingers of the other hand. Push and knead for 36 cycles. For women, knead only with rotatory movements (see Fig. 3).

5. Kneading the whole abdomen: Keep the left hand akimbo with the thumb placed in front of the waist and the other four fingers at the left loin. (This is not required if a lying position is taken.) Move the right palm with a pushing action from the right iliac fossa upwards, passing through the right and left hypochondriac regions and going downwards to the left iliac fossa, and then back to the right iliac fossa, forming a cycle.

Make 18 circles with the right palm. Then repeat the exercise with the left palm in the opposite direction, starting from the left iliac fossa, for another 18 circles (see Fig. 4).

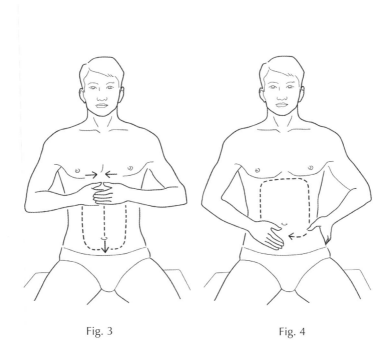

Fig. 3   Fig. 4

6. Digital pressure, palmar pressure and rotation: A combination of these manipulations with kneading may give better results.

Digital pressure is performed by pressing Zhongwan (CV 12), Qihai (CV 6) and Guanyuan (CV 4) with the index and middle fingertips or the index, middle and ring fingertips. Press the fingertips down and gradually raise them. Repeat five to seven times at each point.

Palmar pressure is pressing the loins with the base of the palm. Place the palms on the sides of the waist with the fingertips pointing forward and the thumbs along the lower border of the costal arches. When pressing with the back part of the palm interiorly and anteriorly, the abdomen bulges, and when the pressure is removed, the abdomen bounces back. Repeat the pressing nine times (see Fig. 5).

Rotation is performed while sitting with the legs crossed and the hands placed on the knees. Rotate the upper portion of the body in a circle clockwise nine times and counterclockwise nine times. The size of the circle should be gradually increased (see Fig. 6).

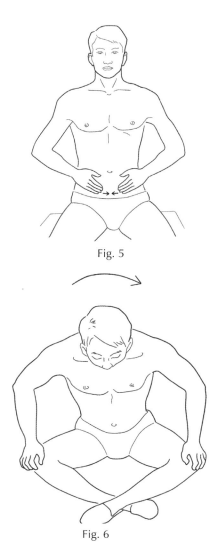

Fig. 5

Fig. 6

III. Frequency of abdomen-kneading

This kneading exercise is usually performed two or three times a day, in the morning and in the evening. At each exercise session, the number of kneading actions can vary depending on the health condition. During the course of an illness, for example, or while experiencing abdominal pain, the number of kneading strokes can be greatly increased until the symptom is relieved. Generally speaking, after kneading one should feel comfortable and relaxed but not fatigued.

Notes

1. During the exercise, breathing should be natural and attention concentrated on where the hand is kneading.

2. Kneading through clothing will not achieve the desired result. It is better to unfasten clothes and knead directly on the abdomen. The manipulations should be gentle, slow and continuous, but not too forceful, to avoid injuring internal organs.

3. During or after kneading, there may be borborygmi, wind breaking, belching, a feeling of warmth inside the abdomen, hunger, or even a desire to defecate or urinate. These are normal reactions to the increased physiological function of the stomach and intestines.

4. During menstruation, the abdomen can be kneaded as usual, except for the lower abdomen, where kneading should be avoided completely or only performed very gently. It is particularly important to be protected from cold during the exercise. Kneading should not be performed when hungry or immediately after a heavy meal. If there is a desire to defecate or urinate, start the exercise after discharge.

Contraindications

Kneading the abdomen is contraindicated during pregnancy. Patients suffering from cancers in the abdomen, gastrointestinal perforation, internal bleeding and peritonitis must not perform kneading. If there is infection of the abodominal wall, kneading of the infected area should be avoided.

8

Treatment of Lower Back Pain
"Back-Moving"

Functional pain of the lower back usually refers to lumbar muscle strain, often occurring in middle-aged and older people. It is characterized by chronic dull pain or soreness aggravated by fatigue. It can be treated with physical therapy. "Back-moving" is an effective physical therapy for exercising the lumbodorsal muscles. It originated from the successive back-moving steps in taiji, a kind of Chinese shadowboxing.

The lower back pain in lumbar muscle strain is chiefly caused by insufficient strength of the lumbar muscles and ligaments and instability of the spinal column. Exercising the lumbodorsal muscles by "back-moving" can increase the strength of the lumbar muscles and the stability and flexibility of the spinal column. Furthermore, the rhythmic contraction and relaxation of the lumbodorsal muscles can improve blood circulation and tissue metabolism in the lumbar regions. Massage Shenshu (B 23) (which is on the lower back, 1.5 cun lateral to the midpoint between the spinous processes of the second and third lumbar vertebrae) with the thumbs to tonify the kidneys, strengthen the waist and alleviate lower back pain (see Fig. 1).

The "back-moving" exercise is simple and suitable for any age. Its frequency and intensity should depend on the individual's age and constitution, and any fatigue felt after the exercise should quickly disappear. The exercise is generally performed twice a day, for about 20 minutes each time. If there is severe pain in the lower back, immediate practice of "back-moving" may have a soothing analgesic effect.

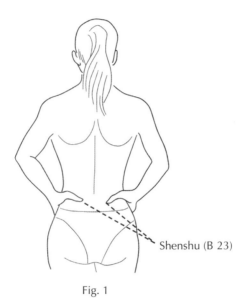

Shenshu (B 23)

Fig. 1

Instructions

There are two types of "back-moving" exercise:

1. "BACK-MOVING" WITH THE ARMS AKIMBO

Preparatory posture: Stand erect with the chest stuck out, the head raised and the eyes looking ahead. Place the hands on the hips, the elbows bent outwards with the thumbs in the back, pressing on Shenshu (B 23), and the four fingers in front.

Movements: Start with the left leg. Raise the left leg backwards as far as possible and take a step back with the body weight moving in the same direction. Allow the anterior part of the left sole to touch the ground first, and then the whole left sole, with the body weight centered on the left leg. Then repeat with the right leg. Alternate stepping back with the left and right legs. During each step back, massage Shenshu (B 23) once with the thumbs. Each step should be about 60 to 70 cm long. Step at a rate of about 40 steps per minute, completing at least 600 steps in 20 minutes (see Fig. 2).

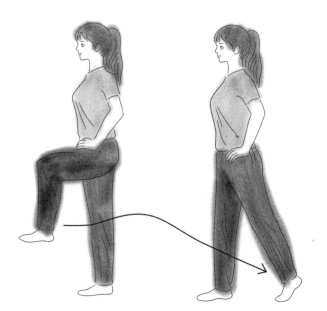

Fig. 2

2. "BACK-MOVING" WITH THE ARMS SWINGING

Preparatory posture: Stand erect with the chest stuck out, the head raised, the eyes looking ahead and the arms hanging down naturally.

Movements: The movements of the legs are the same as in exercise 1. In addition, while moving back, swing the arms as the leg moves. Stick out the chest during the backward movements and raise the leg as far as possible (see Fig. 3).

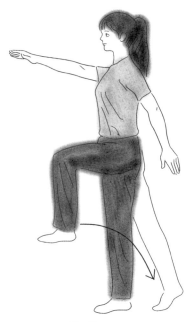

Fig. 3

Notes

1. You may select either of the two types or alternate both types.

2. The ground should be level without any obstacles, or perform the exercise indoors.

3. Organic diseases such as tuberculosis and malignant tumors are contraindications.

4. In an acute case of severe lumbago, the cause of pain should be determined first. Only functional pain of the lower back can be treated with this method.

In addition to lower back pain, hunchback can also be prevented by doing this exercise, which can increase the ability to move backwards and the dorsal extension of the back.

9

Treatment of Sciatica
Lying, Sitting and Standing

The sciatic nerve is located deep in the muscles of the buttocks, originating from the sacral plexus and running distally along the thigh with its branches to the lower leg and foot. It is an important nerve of the lower extremities, for both motor and sensory purposes.

Sciatica is a painful inflammation of the sciatic nerve, usually a neuritis, but it may also result from pressure caused by a tumor or inflammation of the neighbouring bones, tendons or muscles, particularly by a protruding intervertebral disc. In an acute case of protrusion of intervertebral disc, there is a cutting pain that radiates from the iliacsacral region to the foot, causing an inability to walk. When it becomes chronic, the patient will feel a dull stretching pain and have difficulty walking.

To determine the cause is the most important thing in the treatment of sciatica. If the pain is caused by pressure from outside the nerve, the pressure should be relieved. If sciatica is the result of inflammation, bed rest, analgesics, acupuncture and massage therapy are indicated. In chronic cases, the following system of physical therapy is advised.

There is a saying in China: "A door-hinge is never worm-eaten." This means that appropriate motion can prevent strain. Therefore, a patient with sciatica should not stop moving for fear of pain. Remaining motionless will aggravate the symptoms.

In chronic cases of sciatic neuritis, the pain is associated with adhesion around the nerve. "Lying, sitting and standing" is a great treatment for this condition, exercising the sciatic nerve by tightening and relaxing it and helping to relieve adhesion and alleviate pain after repeated practice.

Instructions

1. Lying: Lie supine in the bed with the legs bent. Without allowing the feet to leave the surface of the bed, straighten the legs one after the other. While they are stretched straight, lift the legs above the bed alternately. Lift the healthy leg to an angle of 90 degrees and the affected leg to an angle of 45 degrees at first. By practicing, the affected leg can also be gradually lifted higher to 90 degrees (see Fig. 1).

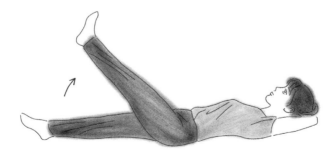

Fig. 1

2. Sitting: Sit upright on a mat or on the floor with the legs straight in front, the feet flexed so that the heels touch the ground and the hands placed flat on the thighs. Gradually reach forward, bending from the lower back while the hands move toward the feet. At first the hands may reach only the shins; but with practice they will be able to reach the toes and the soles of the feet (see Fig. 2).

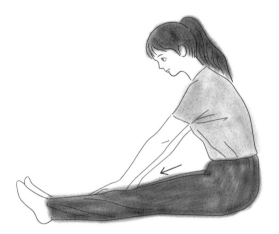

Fig. 2

3. Standing: Stand with the arms akimbo. Raise the left and right leg alternately while keeping it straight. Then stand with the feet as far apart as possible. Bend the left knee and squat down, forming a bow step; repeat, bending the right knee. Bend the left and right knees alternately. This exercise stretches the lower extremity of the unbent side (see Fig. 3).

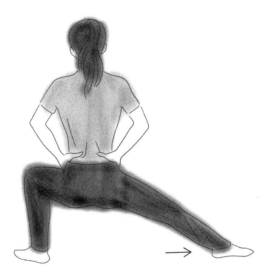

Fig. 3

10

Anus-Lifting Exercise
A Method for Preventing and Treating Hemorrhoids

Hemorrhoids is a common chronic condition, often complicated in more severe cases by prolapse of the rectum, anemia, anal fistula or abscess.

The anus-lifting exercise—that is, constriction of the anus—is a simple, practical method for preventing and treating hemorrhoids. In fact, it was proposed in ancient times and recorded in Zhen Zhong Fang (Formulae under the Pillow), written by the famous physician Sun Simiao early in the Tang Dynasty. It is also one of the key points in either qigong practice or taijiquan exercise.

The pathogenesis of hemorrhoids is closely related to difficulty in backflow of venous blood. Muscular contraction helps the venous blood flow back to the heart. Sitting for long periods, old age, a weak constitution and excessive accumulation of fat in the abdomen are the common factors that cause weakness of the intestinal and perianal muscles, interfering with the venous backflow and leading to venous dilation and congestion at the lower end of the rectum, thereby causing the formation of hemorrhoids. The anus-lifting exercise can strengthen peri-anal muscles to prevent venous dilation. Combining this with breathing exercises can further increase the cardiovascular function and venous backflow to remove rectal and anal congestion. In addition, it can promote intestinal peristalsis and prevent constipation. Thus, the anus-lifting exercise can improve blood circulation of the perianal tissues either to prevent or to cure hemorrhoids.

Four key points are essential to successful anus-lifting: inhaling, touching the palate with the tongue, lifting the anus and holding the breath.

Instructions

Relax the body but tuck the buttocks in and draw the thighs together with force, at the same time inhaling and touching the palate with the tongue. Constrict and lift the anus as if to prevent defecation. After holding the breath for a while, exhale and relax.

This exercise is very simple and can be performed at any time, anywhere and in any posture—sitting, lying or standing. However, it is best to make a timetable for exercise according to specific circumstances, including the time and number of exercises. Generally speaking, perform the exercise at least twice a day (in the morning and in the evening) and for not too long, to prevent fatigue.

Notes

1. This exercise is helpful for internal and external hemorrhoids, prolapse of the rectum and anal fistula, but it is contraindicated if there is severe pain caused by anal fissure, inflammatory hemorrhoids, perianal abscess, incarcerated prolapse of the rectum and other local inflammations.

2. Persevere and do the exercise every day without skipping days.

3. Avoid pungent and other stimulating food.

4. Avoid taking a long time to relieve oneself; in particular, don't read during defecation.

5. Try to eliminate all the causes of hemorrhoids, especially constipation.

6. Other auxiliary remedies can be used in combination with the anus-lifting exercise, such as rinsing the anus with warm water after bowel movements and before going to bed, putting a hot compress on the anus or using perianal massage to promote local blood circulation. The anus-lifting exercise will be even more effective if it is combined with qigong therapy.

11

Waist-Rubbing Exercise

The waist-rubbing exercise is a good form of physical therapy for functional lumbar conditions. The exercise is simple, but the effect remarkable.

The waist-rubbing exercise includes six kinds of movements: rubbing, pinching, massaging, tapping, scratching and rotating.

1. Rubbing: Sit upright with feet shoulder width apart. Rub the palms until they are hot and press them firmly on Yaoyan (Ex-B 7) on both sides of the small of the back (the depressions 3 to 4 cun lateral to the spinous processes of the third lumbar vertebrae) for a period of three to five breaths. Then rub forcefully with the palms along the sides of the lumbar vertebrae up and down from Changqiang (GV 1) (midway between the tip of the coccyx and the anus) to where the arms can be retroflexed. Rub in succession 36 times (see Figs 1 and 2).

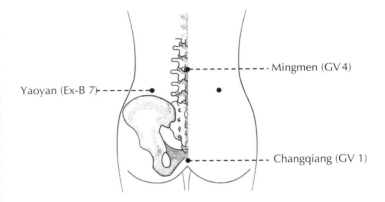

Yaoyan (Ex-B 7)

Mingmen (GV 4)

Changqiang (GV 1)

Fig. 1

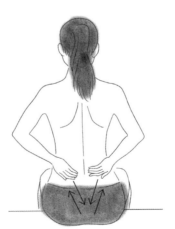

Fig. 2

2. Pinching: Pinch the skin along the midline of the back with the thumb and forefinger of both hands from Mingmen (GV 4) (on the posterior midline of the lower back, in the depression between the spinous processes of the second and third lumbar vertebrae) down to the coccyx by gripping and loosening the grip alternately. Perform four rounds (see Fig. 3).

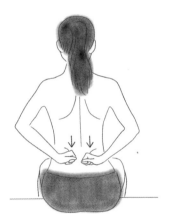

Fig. 3

3. Massaging: Clench the fists gently. With the radial aspect of the fists facing upwards, massage the sides of the small of the back with the prominent parts of the metacarpophalangeal articulation clockwise for 18 circles and counterclockwise for 18 circles. This can be performed on both sides simultaneously or on one side first and then on the other (see Fig. 4).

4. Tapping: Clench the fists gently. With the radial aspect of the fists facing downwards, tap the palmar aspect of the fists on the sacrococcygeal region, causing no pain. Tap 36 times on each side (see Fig. 5).

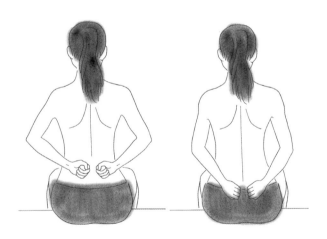

Fig. 4   Fig. 5

5. Scratching: Place the hands on the hips with the elbows pointing outwards and the thumbs in front. Press on the sides of the waist and don't move. Meanwhile, scratch with the palmar aspect of the other fingers from the sides of the lumbar vertebrae outwards on both sides simultaneously 36 times (see Fig. 6). (Cut the nails short beforehand to avoid injuring the skin during scratching.)

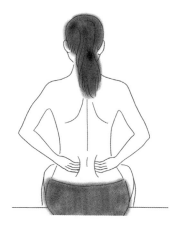

Fig. 6

6. Rotating: Stand upright with the feet shoulder width apart and arms akimbo (thumb in the rear and the fingers in front).

(a) Push forwards with both hands to stick the abdomen out and bend the upper torso back.

(b) Push to the right with the left hand, bending the upper torso to the left as far as possible.

(c) Push backwards with both hands to stick the buttocks out with force and bend the upper torso forwards as far as possible.

(d) Push to the left with the right hand, bending the upper torso to the right as far as possible.

These four actions form a circular movement. Rotate in this way nine times clockwise and nine times counterclockwise (see Fig. 7).

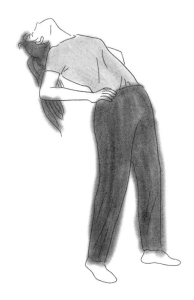

Fig. 7

Notes

1. The rotation of the waist should be slow; rapid and excessive rotation may sprain the lumbus.

2. Generally, the sitting posture is used, but with a low room temperature the exercise can also be performed in bed with the patient lying on his or her side, covered with a quilt. In this case, massage one side first and then the other. The rotating action can be done after getting dressed.

3. For prevention of lower back pain, 36 repetitions of each action are enough; but for therapeutic purposes, the number of repetitions should be increased to 50 or 60 or even more than 100 until sweating starts. However, don't practice too much, to avoid overfatigue.

Why does the waist-rubbing exercise have such a remarkable effect on lower back pain? From a medical point of view, rubbing of the lumbar region causes capillary dilatation, promotes local blood circulation, improves the supply of blood nutrients to the lumbar muscles and accelerates the removal of metabolic products. In this way, the lumbar muscles are developed, prevented from atrophy, and the elasticity and tenacity of ligaments and motility of lumbar vertebral joints are increased. Therefore, the waist-rubbing exercise is effective for preventing and treating functional pain in the lumbar region, especially chronic lumbar muscle strain, acute lumbar sprain and postural lumbago. It can also be used for the treatment of lumbar intervertebral disc protrusion and sciatica.

However, it is absolutely contraindicated in lumbago caused by organic diseases such as tuberculosis, tumor, fracture and bacterial infection of the lumbar vertebrae.

12

Waist-Turning Exercise
A Remedy for Constipation

Habitual constipation is a common ailment, frequently occurring in older people and in patients with chronic diseases or who have just had operations.

The causes of habitual constipation are multifarious, and include prolonged sitting, lack of physical exercise or physical activity, irregular life, no fixed time for bowel movements and insufficient intake of water and food rich in fiber. Among these, long-term lack of exercise is the most serious, because it weakens the muscles involved in defecation (diaphragmatic muscle, abdominal muscles, levator ani muscle) and intestinal peristalsis, so that food residues stay in the intestines too long, and result in excessive absorption of water and formation of hard fecal masses.

Waist-turning is an ancient remedy for habitual constipation. It is easy to practice and is effective.

The exercise is designed to build up the lumbar, abdominal and pelvic muscles, increase the intestinal secretions and enhance gastric and intestinal peristalsis, facilitating defecation. At the same time, it is also good for regulating both the nervous system and gastrointestinal activities, and is therefore effective in curing functional disturbances of the intestines from either constipation or diarrhea.

Instructions

Preparatory posture: Stand with the feet apart, somewhat splaying and spaced at a little more than shoulder width, and with arms akimbo. Keep the body upright, and bend the knees slightly with the knee not beyond the tips of the toes (see Fig. 1).

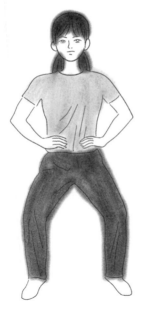

Fig. 1

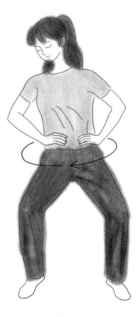

Fig. 2

Movements: Take the umbilicus as the axis and turn the waist and abdomen in the following directions: (1) Turn clockwise from the left, to the front, to the right and then to the back, as shown in Fig. 2 by the arrow. (2) Turn counterclockwise from the right, to the front, to the left and then to the back, as shown in Fig. 3 by the arrow. (3) Imitate the motion of a wheel by moving the waist to the right, downwards, to the left and then upwards, as shown in Fig. 4.

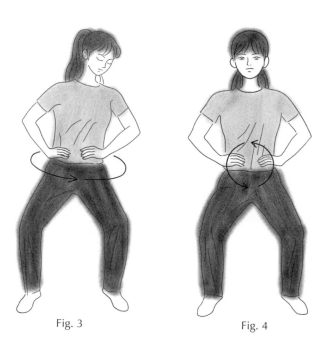

Fig. 3   Fig. 4

(4) Repeat step (3) in reverse, first moving to the left, downwards, to the right and then upwards, as shown in Fig. 5.

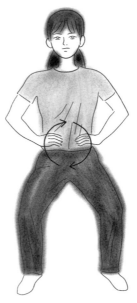

Fig. 5

Notes

1. The chief movements are those of the waist and abdomen, not of the shoulders and knees. The shoulders and knees should be kept motionless or only slightly moved. It may be hard for beginners to avoid turning the upper body while the waist and abdomen is turned but they will master the technique gradually.

2. Do the exercise one to three times a day. The capacity for exercise depends on your constitution and general condition. Generally, you may start with 20 turns in one exercise session and gradually increase to 200 turns. The time spent on each session starts from 30 seconds and increases to about 10 minutes.

3. If you master the first two of these four steps and persevere in practice, you will notice a favourable effect on constipation. If you master all four steps and persevere in practice, not only will habitual constipation or chronic diarrhoea be cured, but the waist and kidneys will also be strengthened.

4. It is preferable to do the exercise early in the morning, before sleep at night or between meals, but not immediately after meals or when you are very hungry. It is important to have a regular lifestyle, to take meals at regular times and to avoid excessive eating and drinking. You are advised to eat food rich in fiber and develop the habit of moving the bowels at a regular time.

5. Do not use this exercise to treat constipation that occurs in case of fever, gastrointestinal tumors, intestinal tuberculosis or discharge of stools with pus and blood. The exercise should be suspended if there is an acute exacerbation of chronic disease or severe dizziness.

6. If this "waist-turning" exercise is practiced in combination with self-massage of the abdomen, the therapeutic effect will be even greater.

13

An Effective Treatment for Enuresis

Enuresis typically occurs in children, but also in young people and even in adults. It is characterized by involuntary discharge of urine during sleep. Although it is not injurious to health, it is often a mental burden and causes inconvenience to the patient and his or her family.

The major cause of enuresis is a functional insufficiency of the kidneys* and urinary bladder so that urination cannot be prevented during sleep. In traditional Chinese medicine, the lumbus is thought to be the seat of the kidneys. Therefore, strengthening the lumbus will enhance the functional activities of the kidneys and urinary bladder, improve the nervous regulation of micturition, and hence cure enuresis.

Consistent practice of a flexion and extension exercise is good for strengthening the lumbus and tonifying the kidneys. Furthermore, the exercise is practiced with the arms akimbo, so that the flexion and extension of the lower back has the effect of

---

* In traditional Chinese medicine, the kidneys and the urinary bladder are closely related in function, with the former controlling the function of the latter.

massaging Belt Vessel Daimai** to control the Kidney Meridian and improve the function of the urinary bladder.

In addition, Zhongji (CV 3), Guanyuan (CV 4), Qihai (CV 6) and Yinjiao (CV 7) are acupoints on the Conception Vessel indicated for treatment of diseases of the urinary system. Pinching the points on the anterior midline of the lower abdomen can reinforce the energy of the Conception Vessel and thus strengthen the urinary bladder.

It has been shown that an exercise with flexion and extension of the lower back together with massage is a simple and effective method for treating enuresis.

I. Flexion and extension exercise method

Preparatory posture: Stand with the back kept straight, the chest stuck out, the arms akimbo, and the feet shoulder width apart (see Fig. 1).

Movements: Bend the upper torso backward (see Fig. 2), and then resume the preparatory posture. Tilt the uppper torso forward as much as possible (see Fig. 3) and then resume the preparatory posture. Repeat the flexion and extension. Generally, practice four times a day, 5 minutes each time. For those with strong constitutions, the exercise may be prolonged appropriately.

** Belt Vessel Daimai is one of the eight extra meridians, originating from the hypochondrium and running transversely around the waist like a belt, performing the function of binding up all the meridians.

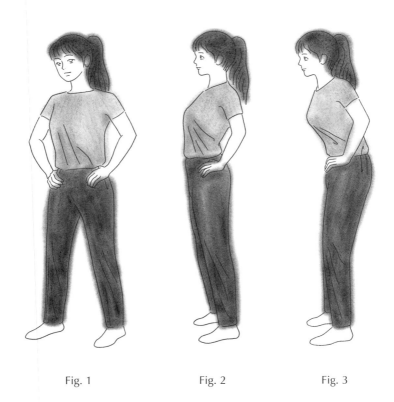

Fig. 1   Fig. 2   Fig. 3

II. Massage method

Lie supine. Pinch and lift the abdominal wall with the right thumb and index finger, starting from the upper border of the symphysis pubis along the anterior midline up to the umbilicus (see Figs 4 and 5). The manipulation can be repeated many times if it causes no pain.

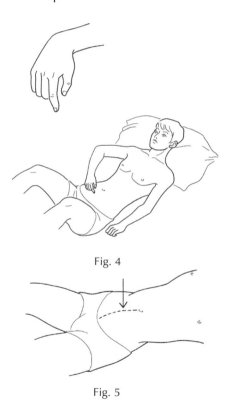

Fig. 4

Fig. 5

For children, parents may perform the manipulation before they go to bed. If the child is uncooperative, the manipulation can be performed during sleep.

Course of treatment: Ten days' treatment constitutes a course. A three-day interval is recommended between courses. A therapeutic effect is usually obtained after four courses. If there is still no obvious improvement, a urological examination is necessary to look for other causes of enuresis.

Notes

1. Determine the exercise load according to the constitution. No obvious fatigue should follow the flexion and extension exercise.

2. The "pinching" action should be performed gently. It is advisable to spread talcum powder on the skin to avoid injuries during pinching.

3. Oxyuriasis, redundant prepuce, anal fissure and constipation should be treated in a timely manner.

4. Train the child to wake up at a regular time during the night to discharge urine.

5. Restrict fluid intake at supper and before sleep. Strenuous exercises and overfatigue should be avoided, as should going to bed at a late hour.

6. Parents' encouragement will give children more confidence and help to achieve the therapeutic effect. Blaming the child will make the child fearful and nervous, interfering with the treatment.

In addition, you could shorten the bed so that the child is forced to lie on his or her side. In such a posture, discharge of urine will immediately stimulate the external sex organs and the inner thigh, promptly waking the child to control urination voluntarily. This approach is considered an auxiliary treatment to the flexion and extension exercise, and sometimes it can cure enuresis in itself.

14

Treatment of Pain in the Knee Joint by Physical Exercise

The knee is one of the big joints that bear the weight of the body and major load in various movements. Walking, standing, sitting, running and jumping all involve this joint. That is why it is so easily injured—for example, in strain caused by excessive movement, sprain as a result of unexpected twisting, knocking or tumbling, and rheumatism resulting from exposure to cold and damp. In all these conditions, it becomes difficult to move the knee joint.

In traditional Chinese medicine it is held that the knee joint is the site where the tendons of the major muscles of the lower extremity congregate. Difficulty in movement of the knee joint or the need to lean on a stick while walking is a sign of failure of the functions of these tendons. Several thousand years ago, the Chinese treated conditions of the knee joint with decoctions, hot medicated compress, acupuncture and physical exercise. In the Jin Dynasty, Chao Yuanfang collected more than 20 kinds of physical exercises for the treatment of conditions of the knee joint in his General Treatise on the Causes and Symptoms of Diseases (610). These exercises have been handed down for more than 1,000 years, and similar ones are still in use at present. The following are some of the simple exercises.

1. Holding the knees close to the chest: Stand erect and relax the whole body. Raising the right leg and bending the knee, hold the knee with both hands and pull it close to the chest. After a while, drop the hands and let the right leg return to its original position. Then raise the left leg and exercise as described above. Repeat 10 to 15 times (see Fig. 1).

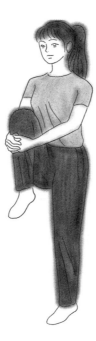

Fig. 1

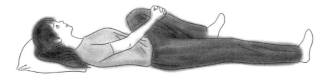

Fig. 2

If there is difficulty in standing during flexion of the knee, take a supine position. Hold the knee with both hands and pull the knee as close to the chest as possible (see Fig. 2).

Consistent practice of this exercise can reduce difficulty in flexion and extension of the knee.

2. Twisting the knees in rotation: Place the legs together and bend the knees to form a half-squatting position. Support the knees with the hands and gently rotate in all directions: clockwise and counterclockwise alternately for 10 to 15 turns. The action should not be too rapid or forceful (see Fig. 3).

This exercise can increase the strength of the ligaments of the knee, which is not only beneficial to the flexion and extension of the knee but also effective for treating chronic rheumatism.

3. Bending knees and squatting: Stand with the legs shoulder width apart. Support the knees with the hands and slowly squat down, moving the buttocks as close to the calves as possible. After staying in this position for a while, gradually stand up. Repeat five to ten times (see Fig. 4).

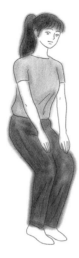

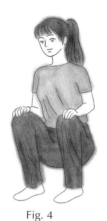

Fig. 4

Fig. 3

This exercise is good for strengthening the muscles of the thigh, especially the quadriceps muscle.

Consistent practice will produce good results and will be even more effective if combined with drug therapy. It should be noted that in the acute stage of injury or rheumatism with swelling and congestion of the knee joint, forced actions are contraindicated. The exercise should be started only when the acute stage is over. Other conditions of the knee joint such as meniscus damage or chondromalacia patellae should only be treated under a doctor's direction.

15

Self-Massage for Insomnia

Insomnia is a distressing symptom. How annoying it is to toss about in bed, unable to sleep. After having a hard time falling asleep, nightmares may ensue, and one may be woken by fright. Sometimes, one is wakeful all night long. In traditional Chinese medicine, insomnia is attributed to the following causes:

1. Excessive mental strain leading to consumption of qi and blood and insufficiency of the heart and spleen.

2. Blood deficiency of the heart, resulting in disturbance of the heart function and mental uneasiness.

3. Psychic depression giving rise to disorders of the liver qi, which interferes with mental activities, including sleeping.

4. Improper diet impairing the spleen and stomach, and a dysharmonious stomach interfering with normal sleep.

In summary, excessive mental strain, anxiety, a weak constitution, irregular diet and impaired digestion can all cause insomnia.

There are many therapies for insomnia in traditional Chinese medicine. One of the simplest therapies is self-massage. Since ancient times, self-massage has been one of the effective ways of maintaining health and preventing disease.

In the Ming Dynasty, Zhang Jiebin cited the following passage from Su's Formulae for Maintaining Health when he discussed health maintenance: "Rub the soles with the hands to raise the qi to the top of the head. Hotness will be felt in the lower abdomen, waist and back. Then rub the corners of the eyes, the ears and nape until they feel hot. Pinch the bridge of the nose five to seven times on the left and then on the right side. Comb the hair a hundred and more times, and then go to bed. You will sleep fast until the morning comes."

Instructions

1. The head: Rub the palms of the hands together until they are hot. Then rub the face with the palms 10 to 20 times. Massage the Yintang (Ex-HN 3), which is located between the eyebrows, with the tip of the middle finger 30 times. Then massage the superciliary ridge along the eyebrow and Taiyang (Ex-HN 5) 30 times, until soreness and distension is felt at the massage point (see Fig. 1).

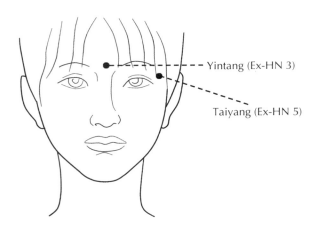

Fig. 1

2. The ears: Massage both ears with the thumb and index finger in a downwards direction 20 times. (Put the thumb on the back of the auricle, and the index finger on the front.) Then rub the earlobes in the same way 30 times until the ears feel hot.

3. The neck: Massage the depression next to the mastoid process behind the ear (Anmian, which literally means "sleeping point") with the index finger, rubbing and kneading 15 times. Then massage with four fingers along the outer side of the sternocleidomastoid muscle from top to bottom 20 times. The massage may be done with strength, but not too fast, until there is a feeling of pressure in the neck (see Fig. 2).

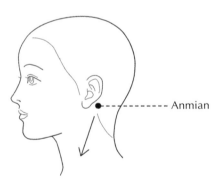

Fig. 2

4. The abdomen: This massage is best practiced before sleep. Take a supine position, rub the palms until they are hot, and massage the abdomen in a clockwise direction with one palm 20 times and then counterclockwise another 20 times. Use the left and right palms alternately. Massaging the abdomen can not only cure insomnia but also strengthen the stomach and promote digestion. It is therefore particularly helpful for insomnia patients with gastric troubles.

5. The center of the sole of the foot: This massage can be done while washing your feet. First, heat your feet including the ankles with hot water (as hot as you can bear). After the feet become red and hyperemic with dilated capillaries, massage the bilateral Yongquan (K 1), the center of the sole of the foot, with the pads of both thumbs 90 times. This can regulate liver function, strengthen the stomach, help induce sleep and promote health (see Fig. 3).

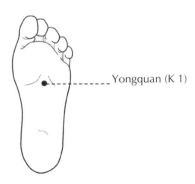

Yongquan (K 1)

Fig. 3

Of the above-mentioned five types of massage, the first three can be done in the daytime, whereas the last two are better performed before sleep. To keep your mind focused and concentrated, count the number of massage strokes as you practice. If you practice self-massage every day, insomnia will be alleviated. Of course, you also have to pay attention to your emotional state, diet and daily life, and avoid overstrain and overfatigue.

16

Massage Treatment for Ménière's Syndrome

Ménière's syndrome is characterized by a sudden onset of vertigo. Its cause is still unknown, but in most cases it is the result of excessive mental strain or overfatigue. According to traditional Chinese medicine, massage of certain areas can promote the circulation of qi and blood, protect the brain and regulate its function. Therefore, such massage may be helpful for the treatment of Ménière's syndrome.

Massage method

Point selection and order of massage: Yintang (Ex-HN 3), Meiyao, Sizhukong (TE 23), Tongziliao (G 1), Taiyang (Ex-HN 5), Shangguan (G 3), Ermen (TE 21), Qubin (G 7) and Chengqi (S 1) (see Fig. 1).

Manipulation:
1. Massage during remission: Massage the points in the order listed above. The key points are Tongziliao (G 1), Taiyang (Ex-HN 5), Shangguan (G 3) and Ermen (TE 21), and more massage should be applied to these points.

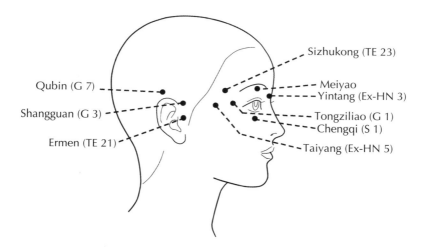

Fig. 1

During massage, keep the eyes gently closed. Make hollow fists with the thumb placed on the middle finger, and stretch out the index finger to press on the point and slowly rub with clockwise turns (see Fig. 2). The mind should be focused and relaxed and the massage action slow with moderate force—not too light and not too heavy. Massage with too light a force is ineffective, and too heavy a force may cause discomfort. Except for Yintang, the points should be massaged on both sides simultaneously. After rubbing, use the index and middle fingers to gently wipe the area from Tongziliao to Taiyang and Shangguan to Ermen several times. Then open your eyes; you will feel clear-headed and comfortable.

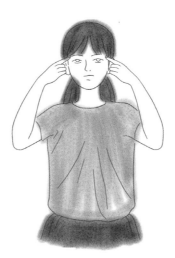

Fig. 2

2. Massage during an attack: If you are having a vertigo attack, massage the key points first, especially Tongziliao (G 1) and Taiyang (Ex-HN 5). If the vertigo is so severe that you are not able to move, you may ask another person to massage you, but the points massaged should be accurate and the force used correct.

It should be noted that this type of massage should be applied immediately after the onset of an attack. In severe attacks, a combination of massage and sedatives is necessary.

A combination of the above massage with massage of the head, eye exercises, ear exercises and appropriate physical exercises may be an excellent way of preventing the recurrence of Ménière's syndrome.

17

Rubbing the Arch of the Foot and Massaging the Head and Neck to Lower Blood Pressure

Hypertension is a common cardiovascular disease. Its main symptoms are headaches and dizziness, which occur in the upper portion of the body. According to traditional Chinese medicine, "disease at the upper should be treated from the lower," so self-massage by rubbing and kneading Yongquan (K 1) in the center of the sole of the foot is helpful for lowering blood pressure. This point has a special function of "bringing down." Rubbing the arch of the foot can bring down the hyperactive fire of the liver and lead blood to flow downwards so that headache and dizziness are alleviated. This is known as "taking away the burning firewood from under the cauldron" or "conducting the fire back to the origin" (origin referring to the lower portion of the body). Furthermore, traditional Chinese medicine holds that massage of the head and neck, especially the hypotensive groove behind the ear and the carotid artery, encourages the blood in the head to flow downwards, thus reducing the uprushing of blood to the head and relieving dizziness and headache.

Since the causes of hypertension are multifarious, its treatment should be complex. However, if self-massage is applied in combination with drug, acupuncture and diet therapies, it will result in a more satisfactory outcome than any of these therapies alone. Self-massage is simple and those suffering from hypertension are advised to try it.

Instructions

1. Rubbing the center of the sole of the foot: Do this daily in the morning before getting up and in the evening before going to sleep. Sit in bed and rub and knead bilateral Yongquan (K 1) (see Fig. 1) with both thumbs a hundred times (about 2 minutes). The center of the sole of one foot can also be rubbed with the heel of the other foot a hundred times. Note that the rubbing should be performed forcefully in the direction of the toes, not to and fro.

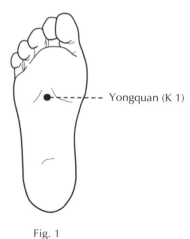

Yongquan (K 1)

Fig. 1

2. Massaging the head and neck: Massage with the palms, starting from the forehead to the vertex and occipital region. Then turn the palms with the fingers directed upward and use the lateral aspect of the fingers to massage the bilateral hypotensive grooves behind the ears (see Fig. 2) and Fengchi (G 20), which is located at the base of the skull, in the depression between the heads of the sternocleidomastoid and trapezius muscles (see Fig. 3). Then move downwards along the sides of the nape and neck to the upper chest while pushing and rubbing the carotid artery with the lateral aspect of the back of the hands. Repeat 10 to 20 times (for about half a minute).

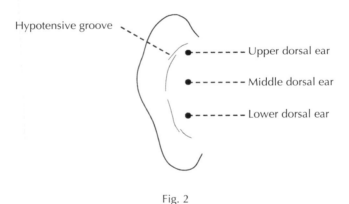

Fig. 2

These two steps can be performed in succession—that is, rubbing the center of the sole of the foot followed by rubbing the head and neck or vice versa. Generally speaking, after the manipulation there will be a comfortable feeling in the head

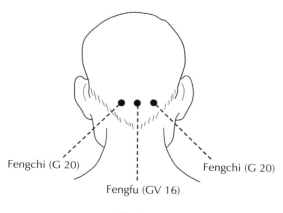

Fengchi (G 20)

Fengchi (G 20)

Fengfu (GV 16)

Fig. 3

and a reduction of the blood pressure by 10–20 mmHg that will last for 4 to 5 hours. To maintain a steady therapeutic effect, massage of the head can be performed at any time.

Although the manipulation is simple, consistent practice is necessary for obtaining a satisfactory result.

Initially, the massage should be combined with drug treatment; the dosage can be gradually reduced under the physician's supervision after the massage treatment begins.

18

Digital Acupoint Pressure for Treating Common Ailments in Older People

A number of ailments frequently occurring in older people can be easily relieved by digital acupoint pressure.

I. Headache

This often results from colds, flu, post-cerebrothrombosis, cerebrovascular spasm and neurosis.

Point selection: Lieque (L 7) is recommended. This is located on the medial aspect of the wrist, 1.5 cun proximal to the wrist crease, immediately superior to the styloid process of the radius (see Fig. 1).

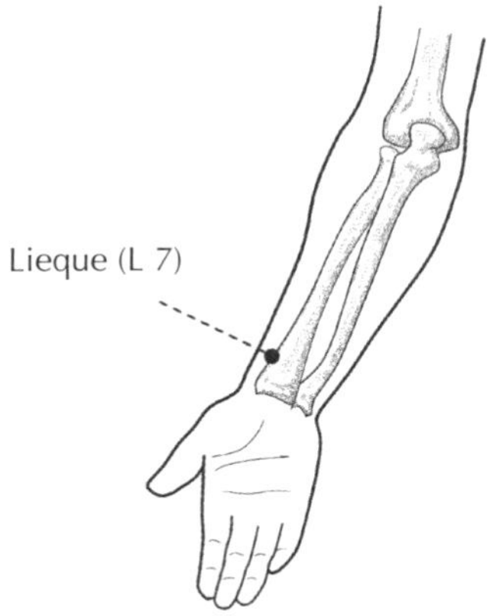

Lieque (L 7)

Fig. 1

Manipulation: Press the point with the radial side of the thumb. Use the point on the right side if the headache is on the left, and the point on the left side if the headache is on the right. If the headache is generalized, use bilateral points. Continuously move the pressing thumb to get the qi—that is, a feeling of soreness and heaviness. About one minute's pressure is necessary for relief of the headache. In addition, combined pressure on bilateral Taiyang (Ex-HN 5) is also recommended (see Fig. 2).

II. Dizziness

This is often caused by Ménière's syndrome, post-concussional syndrome, heatstroke, car sickness and sea sickness.

Point selection: Press Yintang (Ex-HN 3), the midpoint between the eyebrows (see Fig. 2).

Taiyang (Ex-HN5)   Yintang (Ex-HN3)

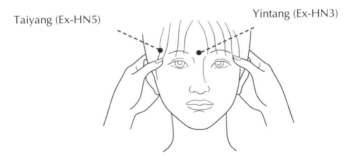

Fig. 2

Manipulation: Press the point with the tip of the index finger or middle finger. Move the fingertip horizontally to get the qi—that is, a feeling of soreness and heaviness in the face. Combined pressure on Shuigou (Renzhong) (GV 26) and Baihui (GV 20) may yield better results.

III. Toothache

Sometimes intolerable toothache is caused by dental cavities, gingivitis, exposure of the dental nerve and other inflammations of the oral cavity.

Point selection: Hegu (LI 4) is recommended. This is located on the dorsum of the hand at the fork of the first and second metacarpal bones (see Fig. 3).

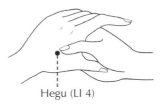

Hegu (LI 4)

Fig. 3

Manipulation: Press the point with a thumb. Move the thumb from the center outwards while tapping the upper and lower teeth together at the same time until the toothache is relieved. Press Hegu (LI 4) on the right for a toothache of the left side, Hegu (LI 4) on the left for a toothache of the right side, and bilateral Hegu (LI 4) for a bilateral toothache. In addition, pressure on Jiache (S 6) may be used when there is pain in the upper teeth (see Fig. 4).

IV. Tinnitus

This is often distressing, both interfering with work and leading to insomnia. Its causes are multifarious, and may be local or general. Acute and chronic otitis media, brain trauma, concussion and Ménière's syndrome are often accompanied by tinnitus in older people.

Point selection: Tinggong (SI 19) is recommended. This is located in the depression in front of the ear and bulges while the teeth are being tapped (see Fig. 4).

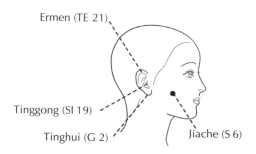

Ermen (TE 21)

Tinggong (SI 19)

Tinghui (G 2)

Jiache (S 6)

Fig. 4

Manipulation: Press Tinggong (SI 19) with the thumb. Pressure on Ermen (TE 21) and Tinghui (G 2) may be applied in combination (Ermen is about 0.6 cun above Tinggong, and Tinghui is 0.6 cun below Tinggong; see Fig. 4). In addition, a kind of massage called "sounding the heaven's drum" can be applied: Alternately cover and uncover the ears with the palms, or insert the index fingers into both external auditory canals at the same time, and move the fingers as if tightening a screw.

19

Treatment of Headache, Syncope, Lumbago, Angina Pectoris and Nocturnal Emission by Digital Acupoint Pressure

Digital acupoint pressure, the process of putting pressure on a given point with the fingertip or fingernail, can be used for treating some common conditions.

I. Treating headache by pressing Taiyang (Ex-HN 5)

Many diseases may lead to headaches. It is of primary importance to find out the cause of a headache. As a symptomatic treatment, digital pressure of Taiyang (Ex-HN 5) is often effective, especially when the headache occurs when you are away from home. Sit upright and keep the neck straight. Press Taiyang hard with one thumb and Fengfu (GV 16) with the other thumb until the headache is relieved. (Taiyang is located in the depression lateral to the external canthus of the eye, and Fengfu is in the depression just below the occipital protuberance; see Figs 1 and 2.)

II. Treating syncope by pressing Renzhong (GV 26)

Syncope is a momentary loss of consciousness caused by temporary ischemia or anoxia of the brain. It is often accompanied by dizziness, blurred vision, nausea, vomiting, sweating, pallor, lowered blood pressure and abnormal pulse (usually rapid at first, then becoming thready and slow, or even leading to transient cardiac arrest).

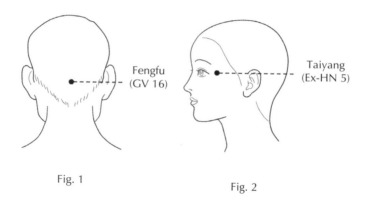

Fengfu
(GV 16)

Taiyang
(Ex-HN 5)

Fig. 1

Fig. 2

Emergency treatment: Lay the patient flat in a well-ventilated place, lower his or her head and undo the collar. Press Renzhong (Shuigou) (GV 26) as well as Hegu (LI 4). (Renzhong is located a third of the way down the philtrum, and Hegu at the fork of the thumb and index finger.) In general, use the thumb or index finger. Bend the first phalangeal joint, and press hard with the fingertip on Renzhong (GV 26). Vibrate the finger to strengthen the pressure and enhance the stimulation. At the same time, pinch Hegu (LI 4) with the nails of the thumb and index finger of the other hand. Continue pressing until the patient regains consciousness (see Figs 3 and 4).

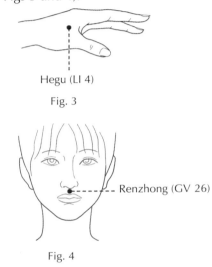

Hegu (LI 4)

Fig. 3

Renzhong (GV 26)

Fig. 4

III. Treating acute lumbar sprain by pressing Weizhong (B40)

Acute lumbar sprain often occurs after suddenly twisting or bending the back or turning the body. It is characterized by severe lumbago and board-like stiffness of the lumbar region with difficulty walking or even the inability to walk. Sometimes even a minute movement of the lumbar region may cause a shooting pain like an electric shock.

Acute lumbar sprain can be treated by pressing Weizhong (B 40). Let the patient lie prone with the legs stretched forwards. Weizhong (B 40) is located in the center of the popliteal crease. Press Weizhong (B 40) forcefully using the pad of the right thumb. The nail should be cut flat beforehand. Ask the patient to shout at the same time. Repetition of the digital pressure is often followed by relief of lumbago and free movement of the back (see Fig. 5).

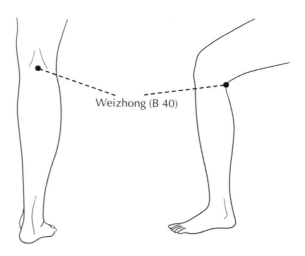

Weizhong (B 40)

Fig. 5

IV. Treating angina pectoris by pressing Neiguan (P 6)

The pain of angina pectoris is characteristically a gripping, boring or pressing sensation in the substernal region or left chest with radiation to the left upper arm. A number of drugs, such as nitroglycerin, are effective in preventing and treating this disease. If an attack occurs unexpectedly, however, and you have no drug with you, press the left Neiguan (P 6) forcefully with the nail-tip of the right thumb until the pain is relieved. Digital pressure of Hegu (LI 4) may be used in combination. (Neiguan is located 2 cun above the wrist crease between the tendons of the palmaris longus and flexor carpi radialis muscles; see Fig. 6.)

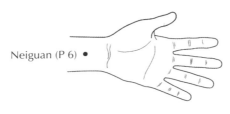

Neiguan (P 6) ●

Fig. 6

V. Treating nocturnal emission by pressing Huiyin (CV 1)

Nocturnal emission can be classified into two types: one is emission during dreaming sleep, and the other is emission during sleep without dreams. If nocturnal emission persists, there will be listlessness, dizziness, tinnitus, loss of memory, lassitude, soreness in the loins and legs, cardiac palpitation and shortness of breath, which interfere with work and study and impair physical and mental health.

Digital pressure of Huiyin (CV 1): Huiyin (CV 1) is located in the perineal region, halfway between the anus and the scrotum. Take a supine position with the legs bent and apart, so that the point is exposed and convenient for digital pressing (see Fig. 7). Press the point with the tip of the middle finger of the right hand, inducing a complex sensation of numbness, distension and soreness. Continue pressing for 1 to 2 minutes.

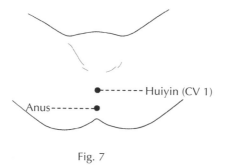

Fig. 7

The above-mentioned five types of digital acupoint pressure are "tricky moves" of traditional Chinese medicine. They can be used either as self-preventive measures or as therapeutic measures for patients. Though simple, digital acupoint pressure can give an immediate cure if it is applied properly.

20

Prevention and Treatment of Systremma (Cramp in the Leg)

Systremma is cramp in the muscles of the calf of the leg, usually occurring in anemic patients, in persons with weak constitutions, after excessive vomiting and diarrhea in acute gastroenteritis, and during exposure to cold. In traditional Chinese medicine, deficiency of qi and blood is considered to be the interior cause, and exposure to cold and wind the exterior cause. The former results in derangement of the muscles, and the latter induces cramps in the muscles. Since the limbs are likely to be attacked by cold and wind, the cramp usually occurs in the limbs, especially in the legs.

I. Limb-extension exercise

There are many methods used to prevent and treat systremma, among which the "limb-extension" exercise is the simplest and easiest. It is recorded in the General Treatise on the Causes and Symptoms of Diseases, compiled by Chao Yuanfang *et al.* in 610, and can be described as follows:

1. Lie supine, extend the arms and legs with the heels apart and the tips of the toes touching one another (see Fig. 1). The limbs are extended as much as possible with effort, and so are the muscles of the toes with the heels apart and the toes touching one another.

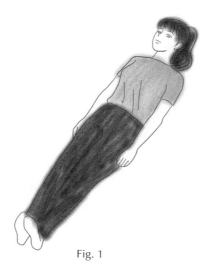

Fig. 1

2. The extension of the limbs is accompanied by breathing. Inhale deeply through the nose and then slowly exhale. Inhale and exhale seven times.

This exercise is aimed at stretching the muscles of the limbs, so there seems to be no substantial movement. However, if it is performed with effort, it is a good exercise of the muscles of the limbs. Do the exercise one to three times a day, and repeat the actions five to ten times at each session. Consistent practice can not only prevent systremma but also drive away any cold sensation in the knees and pain in the calf. This exercise is especially suitable for cramp experienced by patients with weak constitutions or deficiency of qi and blood and for older people.

II. Limb-extension exercise for cramp with intolerable pain

If cramp in the calf is accompanied by intolerable pain, limb-extension can also produce relief. It is also recorded in the General Treatise on the Causes and Symptoms of Diseases and can be described as follows:

1. Putting up with the pain, extend the cramped leg and toes with effort. If the leg cannot be extended straight, press it with both hands or with the other leg (see Fig. 2). The hand can be used to hold the cramped toes straight (see Fig. 3).

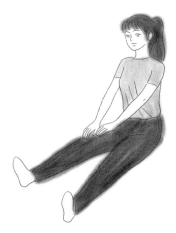

Fig. 2

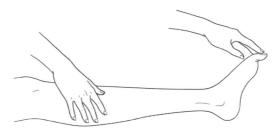

Fig. 3

2. Extension of the cramped limb is accompanied by forcible exhalation together with the sound "heh, heh." The exhalation should be short and rapid with effort, after a full inhalation.

3. To obtain better results, other manipulations can be performed in combination with limb-extension, such as tapping the affected area (tapping the calf if there is systremma; tapping the lateral muscles of the lower leg if there is a cramp in the toes) or massaging Chengshan (B 57), an acupoint located in the posterior aspect of the leg, between the two heads of the gastrocnemius muscle (see Fig. 4).

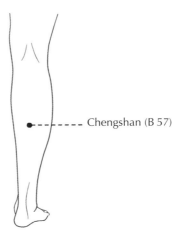
Chengshan (B 57)

Fig. 4

This manipulation can also be used as an emergency treatment of systremma occurring during sports or swimming. If systremma is a result of anemia, reduction of blood calcium or loss of fluid after excessive vomiting and diarrhea, treatment of the primary cause is necessary.

21

Qigong Therapy for Nocturnal Emission, Hemorrhoids and Incontinence of Urine

In older people with weak constitutions, spermatorrhea, hemorrhoids, anal fistula and incontinence of urine are common. In young men, habitual masturbation may lead to frequent nocturnal emission, impairing both physical and mental health. Elevation of the perineum is a qigong therapy that can be effective for treating these conditions.

The perineum is the area between the anus and the genital organs. Perineum elevation refers to the gentle elevation of qi that puts the anus, urethra and the musculature of this area in a state of contraction (as if making effort to avoid releasing stools or urine). The purpose of elevating the perineum is to lead the qi by will, and establish communication between the qi inhaled and the qi elevated to tonify the kidneys and arrest spontaneous emission. From the modern medical point of view, elevating the perineum consistently and consciously improves the blood circulation and nutritional state of the perineal tissue, accentuating the dilating, contracting and restraining functions of the anal sphincter, vesical sphincter and musculature of the sex organs. That is why this therapy is useful for nocturnal emission, spermatorrhea, impotence, premature ejaculation, hemorrhoids, anal fistula, prolapse of the rectum and incontinence of urine.

This kind of qigong therapy has four forms.

I. Supine form

1. Lie supine on a high pillow. Extend the legs and place the feet together. Place the arms and hands naturally alongside the body.

2. Let the tip of the tongue touch the palate. Gently close the eyes and the mouth. Concentrate on Dantian (3 cun below the umbilicus) and empty the mind of all distractions. After saliva begins flowing in the mouth, inhale through the nose and, leading the qi by will, gently elevate the perineum. At the same time, grit the teeth while clenching the fists, flexing the toes forward and downward with force and holding the breath for 3 to 5 seconds. Then gently take the tongue away from the palate, exhaling slowly through the nose and relaxing the whole body naturally.

3. Let the tongue touch the palate again and repeat the actions as described above. Practice for 5 to 10 minutes each time, three times a day (in the morning, at noon and in the evening). The supine form of perineum elevation is effective for nocturnal emission, spermatorrhea, impotence, premature ejaculation and incontinence of urine.

II. Strolling form

1. Walk unhurriedly in a leisurely way. Close the mouth gently, with the tongue touching the palate and the teeth slightly gritted. Concentrate on Dantian and empty the mind of all distractions.

2. Drop the hands down naturally, with the fingers slightly flexed in opposition to the thumb, thus forming hollow fists. Also slightly flex the toes, as if to grip the ground. Then walk slowly and gently elevate the perineum.

3. After strolling for 3 to 5 minutes, slowly relax the perineum. Stroll for another 1 to 2 minutes, and then repeat the above-mentioned actions. Continue exercising for about half an hour, twice a day (in the morning and in the evening before sleep).

The strolling form of perineum elevation is effective for hemorrhoids, anal fistula, prolapse of the rectum and incontinence of urine.

III. Standing form

1. Stand with the legs apart and feet parallel but shoulder width apart. Grip the ground with the toes, bend the knees slightly, relax the waist and hips, keep the upper torso upright and assume a squatting position.

2. Tuck the chin in lightly, relax the chest and drop the arms naturally, with the fingers slightly bent in opposition to the thumb to form hollow fists.

3. Drop the upper eyelids, slightly shut the mouth and gargle with saliva three to five times. Lick the palate and mandible with the tongue and touch the palate with the tip of the tongue until the mouth is full of saliva. Swallow the saliva and touch the palate again with the tongue; then inhale through the nose. Meanwhile, gently elevate the perineum, leading the qi upwards by will along the midline of the back to the vertex, and then to under the tongue. Finally, exhale slowly and relax the perineum. Repeat the above-mentioned actions more than 20 times, and then press on Dantian with the hands overlapping (the left hand below the right hand). Concentrate on Dantian for a while, and then take an unhurried walk for 30 to 50 steps.

This form can be practiced twice a day (in the morning and in the evening) and is effective for the prevention and treatment of the above-mentioned conditions.

IV. Sitting form

Sit on a chair or a bench with the thighs horizontal and the upper torso upright. Clench the fists and place them on the thighs just above the knees. Drop the eyelids and slightly close the mouth. Let the tongue touch the palate. Then perform the same actions as for the standing form. After the exercise, stand up and take a walk at a slow pace for 30 to 50 steps.

This form should also be practiced twice a day (in the morning and in the evening) and sometimes with an additional practice at noon. It is also effective for the above-mentioned conditions.

Part Two

Methods of Keeping Fit

22

Patting All over the Body

Patting all over the body is a simple health-protecting exercise characterized by giving light blows with one's own palms or fists. It is good for strengthening the tendons and bones, facilitating the development of muscles, improving articular motion, accelerating blood circulation and promoting the function of internal organs and metabolism. After patting, one will feel relaxed, quick in action, clear-headed and high-spirited. This kind of health-protecting exercise is more effective than massage by others.

Patting is usually performed with the hands, but sometimes with a steel-wire bat or sandbag. The exercise consists of eight steps.

I. Patting the head

Instructions: Perform this exercise while standing or walking. If standing, relax the whole body, drop the shoulders and elbows, and smile while patting without moving. If walking, saunter while patting at the same time. Pat the left side of the head with the left palm and the right side of the head with the right palm, from the front of the head to the back, to and fro, 50 times. Then pat the lateral parts of the head with both palms

50 times. Count the number of pats silently. The mind should be concentrated and the breath natural (see Figs 1 and 2).

Indications: Prevention and treatment of dizziness, headache and cerebral ischemia.

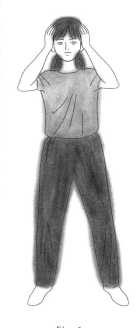
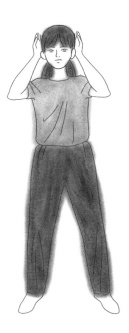

Fig. 1   Fig. 2

II. Patting the arms

Instructions: Stand or walk as described in Step I. Pat the anterior, posterior, lateral and medial aspects of the left arm with the right palm or fist, 25 blows on each aspect (divided into five series of five blows each). Then pat the right arm with the left palm or fist in the same way (see Figs 3 and 4).

Indications: Prevention and treatment of muscular dysplasia of the arm, acrocyanosis, numbness of the arm and hemiplegia.

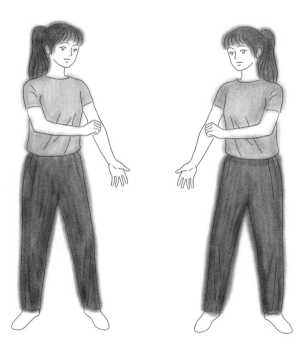

Fig. 3   Fig. 4

III. Patting the shoulders

Instructions: Stand or walk as described in Step I. Pat the left shoulder with the right palm, and then the right shoulder with the left palm. Pat both shoulders alternately 50 to 100 times (see Figs 5 and 6).

Indications: Prevention and treatment of periarthritis of the shoulder, stiffness of the shoulder, muscular dysplasia and atelectasis.

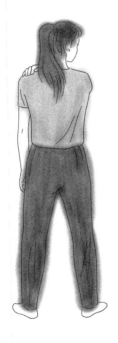
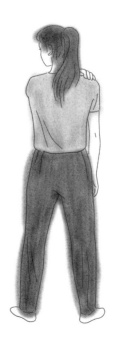

Fig. 5   Fig. 6

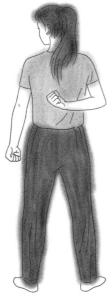
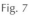

Fig. 7

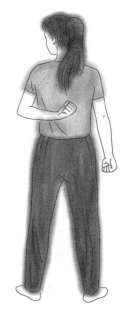

Fig. 8

IV. Patting the back

Instructions: Stand or walk as described in Step I. Pat the left side of the back with the right fist, and then the right side of the back with the left fist, 100 to 200 times on each side (see Figs 7 and 8).

Indications: Back pain, chronic bronchitis, emphysema, atelectasis, muscular dysplasia and coronary heart disease.

V. Patting the chest

Instructions: Pat the left and right sides of the chest alternately, the left side with the right palm or right fist, and then the right side with the left palm or left fist. Pat from the top to the bottom, and then from the bottom to the top, 100 to 200 times on each side (see Figs 9 and 10).

Indications: Coronary heart disease, hypertensive heart disease, rheumatic heart disease, emphysema, atelectasis, pulmonary heart disease, muscular dysplasia.

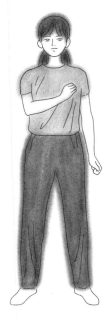

Fig. 9

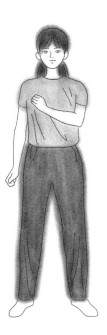

Fig. 10

VI. Patting the waist and abdomen

Instructions: Using the waist as an axis, turn the upper torso to the left and then to the right, pushing the arms forwards. Pat the left side of the abdomen with the right hand and the right side of the abdomen with the left hand, and pat the right side of the waist with the left hand and the left side of the waist with the right hand. Pat the upper and lower parts of the abdomen and the upper, middle and lower parts of the waist 100 to 200 times on each side (see Figs 11 and 12).

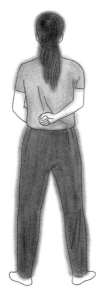

Fig. 11

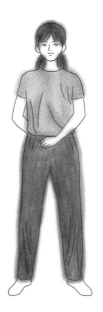

Fig. 12

Indications: Prevention and treatment of soreness in the loins, lumbago, hyperosteogeny, dyspepsia, abdominal distension, constipation.

VII. Patting the buttocks

Instructions: Pat the left side of the buttocks with the left palm or left fist and the right side of the buttocks with the right palm or right fist 50 to 100 times on each side (see Fig. 13).

Indications: Prevention and treatment of dysplasia of the gluteal muscles.

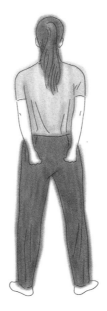

Fig. 13

VIII. Patting the legs

Instructions: Stand with the left leg raised and bent into a right angle at the knee. Place the left heel on a rail. Pat the anterior, posterior, lateral and medial aspects of the thigh and lower leg with the left palm or left fist from the top of the leg downwards 100 to 200 times. Pat the right leg in the same way with the right palm or right fist (see Figs 14 and 15).

Indications: Prevention and treatment of muscular dysplasia of the leg, hemiplegia, paraplegia, acrocyanosis of the lower extremities, numbness and weakness of the leg.

Notes: The patting should be light at first and then gradually become stronger. It will be effective only if the exercise is performed consistently.

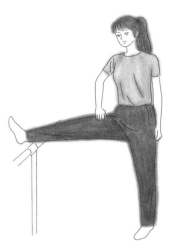

Fig. 14

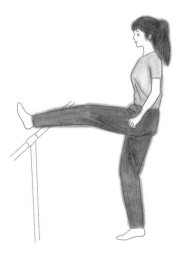

Fig. 15

23

Ten-Minute Self-Massage Before Sleep

A 10-minute self-massage before sleep based on traditional Chinese medical theory is a kind of health-protecting method to improve the constitution and prevent disease. It can also be used as an auxiliary treatment of chronic diseases, being particularly effective for neurasthenia, backache, arthralgia, intercostal neuralgia and aversion to cold during sleep in winter with cold feet all night.

This health-protecting method is simple and can be learned quickly. It does not take much time to practice and its effect is usually satisfactory.

In practicing the 10-minute self-massage, a gentle and repetitive manipulation is applied for the purpose of promoting the circulation of qi and blood in the meridians and collaterals and inducing relaxation. Repeated rubbing of the palms on the massaged areas produces heat and electricity that are conducted into the interior of the body. These dilate the capillaries, improve blood circulation and promote metabolism.

The massage consists of 12 steps:

1. Rubbing Baihui (GV 20): Massage Baihui (GV 20) (located at the vertex, the midpoint of the line extending over the vertex

joining the apexes of the auricles) with rotatory movements 50 times, drawing circles with diameters ranging from 3–5 cm, either clockwise or counterclockwise. The massage lasts for about 30 seconds (see Fig. 1).

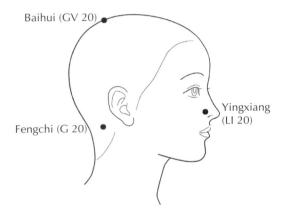

2. Massaging the face: Cover the face with the hands and rub it up and down 50 times for about 30 seconds (see Fig. 2).

3. Kneading Yingxiang (LI 20): Poke and knead bilateral Yingxiang (LI 20) (located in the nasolabial fold, 0.5 cun lateral to the alanasi) with the tips of both index fingers 50 times for about 20 seconds (see Fig. 3).

4. Pushing the ears: Cover the ears with the palms, push the auricles forward to cover the earholes and then push them backwards 50 times for about 30 seconds (see Fig. 4).

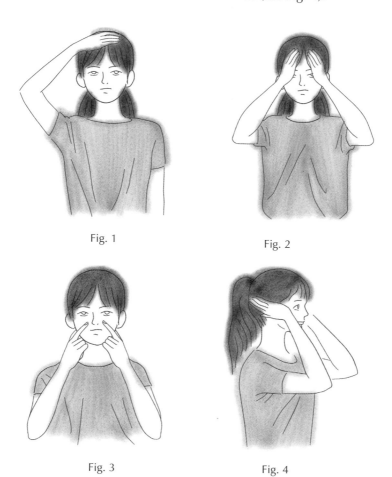

Fig. 1

Fig. 2

Fig. 3

Fig. 4

5. Kneading Fengchi (G 20): Knead bilateral Fengchi (G 20) (located at the base of the skull, in the depression between the heads of the sternocleidomastoid and trapezius muscles) with the index and middle fingers 50 times for about 20 seconds (see Fig. 5).

6. Kneading Jianjing (G 21): Press and knead the left Jianjing (G 21) (located in the depression of the trapezius, superior to the superior angle of the scapula) with the right index and middle fingers 50 times, and then the right Jianjing (G 21) with the left index and middle fingers 50 times, taking 30 seconds for both shoulders (see Fig. 6).

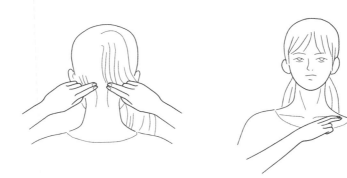

Fig. 5   Fig. 6

7. Massaging the chest and abdomen: Press Qihai (CV 6) (located on the anterior midline, at the midpoint of the superior two-fifths of the line joining the upper border of the symphysis pubis and the umbilicus) with the left palm and Tanzhong (CV 17) (at the midpoint between the nipples) with the right palm. Move the right hand in an arc to Qihai (CV 6) while massaging, and at the same time move the left hand upwards in an arc to Tanzhong (CV 17) while massaging. Then turn back along the same paths. Repeat 50 times for about 30 seconds (see Fig. 7).

8. Massaging the back: Clench the hands into fists and place the back of the fists on the lower back with the pressed points spaced 5 cm to 7 cm apart, corresponding to bilateral Dachangshu (B 25). Move the fists directly upwards as far as possible while massaging forcefully. Unfold the fists and repeat the massage from the lower back 50 times for about 30 seconds (see Fig. 8).

9. Massaging the arms: Stretch the left arm straight with the palm facing down. Press the left arm with the right hand near the acromion and move the right hand distally along the lateral aspect of the left arm to the back of the left hand (see Fig. 9). Then rotate the left wrist outwards with the inner aspect of the arm and the palm facing up, and move the right hand proximally along the inner aspect to the left axilla (see Fig. 10). Repeat 50 times and then massage the right arm the same way 50 times. The manipulation lasts for 2 minutes.

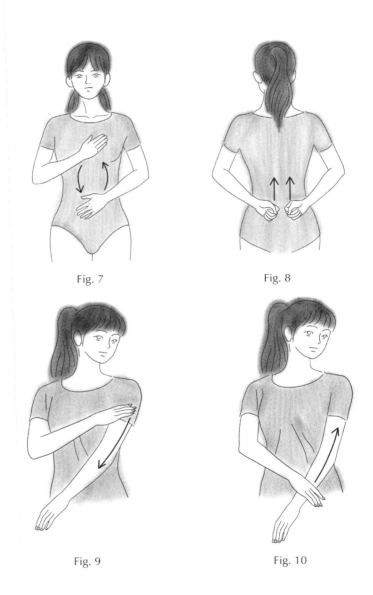

Fig. 7

Fig. 8

Fig. 9

Fig. 10

10. Rubbing the legs: Stretch the legs straight and keep the feet shoulder width apart. Massage the legs with both hands from the hip joints distally along the lateral aspect of the legs to the top of the feet (see Fig. 11), and then massage proximally along the inner aspect of the leg from the arch of the feet to the groin (see Fig. 12). Repeat 50 times for about 2 minutes.

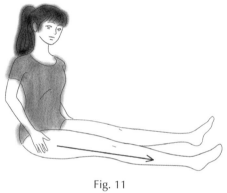

Fig. 11

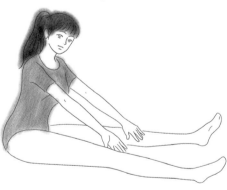

Fig. 12

11. Rubbing the arch of the foot: Rub the sole of the left foot with the right middle finger together with the index and ring fingers, starting from the back part of the sole below the inner ankle and rapidly pushing forwards to Yongquan (K 1) (located in the center of the sole of the foot between the second and third metatarsals, or in the depression formed when the toes are plantar-flexed) (see Fig. 13). Repeat 50 times. Then rub the arch of the right foot with the left hand. The manipulation on both feet takes 30 seconds.

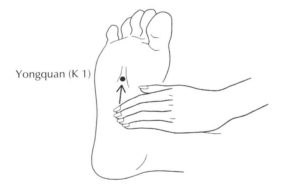

Yongquan (K 1)

Fig. 13

12. Massaging the scrotum in male and breasts in female: For a male, take a supine position, enclose the scrotum with the left hand and massage it in 50 circular movements clockwise. Then massage it with the right hand in 50 circular movements counterclockwise. The total manipulation takes about

40 seconds. For a female, take a supine position, cup one breast with each hand and massage both breasts simultaneously in 50 circular movements, taking about 20 seconds.

Notes

1. Wash the face and feet or take a bath before going to bed and performing the exercise in bed. If the room is warm, take off all clothing except underwear. If it is cool, the massage can be performed with the underclothes on.

2. During the massage, the eyes should be gently shut, the mind concentrated and the tip of the tongue should be touching the palate. The palms should maintain close contact with the skin and the massage should be performed in succession with moderate force. There should be a feeling of warmth all over the body or mild sweating after the whole exercise is completed.

3. When Yingxiang (LI 20), Fengchi (G 20) and Jianjing (G 21) are massaged, force should be exerted to induce a feeling of soreness and distension. When the back is massaged, a short break is allowed to restore the strength of the arms.

4. During the massage of the scrotum, stimulation of the penis should be avoided. For beginners who have not grasped the correct manipulation, erection may occur or even persist. Press Guanyuan (CV 4) (on the anterior midline, two-fifths of the way

superior to the upper border of the symphysis pubis) with the middle finger and gradually increase the pressure. The erection may thus be diminished in 2 minutes.

5. Cold and wind should be avoided in the winter.

6. The time required for each manipulation as mentioned above is only given for beginners. Those familiar with the manipulation do not have to note the time from one manipulation to another. The whole exercise usually takes about 10 minutes.

7. This kind of self-massage is contraindicated in pregnancy, fever and other serious diseases. It is also not recommended if there is skin disease, tumor or infection on the areas of massage.

24

Ten-Minute Qigong Practice

For those who are busy with work and household chores and have little spare time but wish to do some health exercise, the following qigong practice takes only about 10 minutes or less. Of course, if time permits, it is better to practice for 30 minutes.

In the beginning, a secluded place is necessary; after becoming accustomed to the practice, however, it can be performed without disturbance anywhere, even in noisy circumstances.

I. Forms

The practice can be generally classified into three forms: standing, sitting and lying. Beginners may select a form most comfortable and natural for them according to their own habits and customs. The form selected is not crucial.

1. Standing form: Stand with feet shoulder width apart, legs bent and buttocks drawn in, as if gripping a basketball between the knees. The exercise load of the lower extremities depends on the extent to which the legs are bent. Extend the hands forwards in front of the chest with the palms facing each other, fingers apart, arms bent in an arc, shoulders rounded and elbows dropped, as if getting ready to catch a flying basketball.

2. Sitting form: Sit upright or take a semi-reclining position with the legs and knees shoulder width apart as if gripping a basketball between the knees. Extend the hands forwards in front of the chest with the palms facing each other, fingers apart, arms bent in an arc, shoulders rounded and elbows dropped, as if holding a basketball. The exercise load depends on the extent of the bend in the arms. The more the arms are extended forwards, the greater the exercise load. If strength is lacking, the upper arms may hang down along the sides of the body, the elbows bent to an angle of 90 degrees and the forearms extended straight forward.

3. Lying form: This form of the exercise, if practiced before sleep, has a marked effect on treating insomnia. Extend the arms straight above the head with the palms facing each other, fingers apart. If there is sufficient muscular strength, raise the arms diagonally behind the head, forming an obtuse angle between the arm and the supine body. The hands are shoulder width apart. If there is an extremely remarkable "feeling of qi" during practice, the arms may be extended outwards. The further apart the hands are, the greater the exercise load.

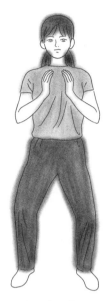

Standing form

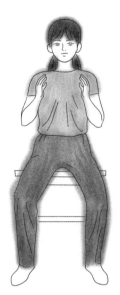

Sitting form

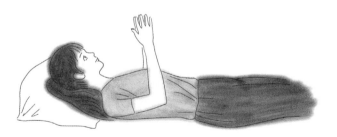

Lying form

II. Action

Open and close the palms. Open means moving the palms apart, and close means moving them towards each other. When a sitting form is taken, the knees can also be opened and closed. There are four categories of opening and closing actions based on the extent of movement: extensive, moderate, minute and no action. The action of the palms and that of the knees should be done separately or alternately to avoid distractions.

III. Mind

1. Opening and closing actions in the mind: This is not a real action but only the recall of actions in the mind. To recall the actions in the mind is the most fundamental point of qigong practice.

2. Resisting power in the mind: While doing the opening and closing actions, a thought of resistance should be kept in mind—imagine a big balloon, a spring or a rubber band between the palms or knees resisting against the actions. This resisting power in the mind can give a balance exercise to the efferent and afferent pathways and to the sensory and motor centers. It is the fundamental condition for producing the feeling of qi and promoting its circulation along the meridians and collaterals.

Instructions

First, perform the opening and closing actions, which may be synchronized with respiration (actions with larger amplitude) or with the pulse (actions with smaller amplitude). Practice starting with extensive movements, gradually changing to minute movements, and accentuate the concentration to perceive the minute actions so that the mind will enter the state of tranquility naturally. Then recall the opening and closing actions in the mind with no physical movement—that is, the body is still while the mind is in action, or motion exists in stillness.

During practice, physical actions and the actions in the mind may proceed in alternation or in combination, making the exercise full of changes. There seems to be a magnetic attraction or a feeling of pulling by a rubber band between the palms when they are being "opened." This is called "closing existing in opening." Similarly, there seems to be a feeling of magnetic expulsion or the existence of a mass of air between the palms when they are being "closed." This is called "opening existing in closing." In addition, several closing actions in the mind may be added to the extensive actions of opening, and several opening actions in the mind may be added to the extensive actions of closing. During the practice with only actions in the mind, the change in the feeling of qi can induce involuntary opening and closing actions of the palms.

Ten-minute qigong practice can improve the ability to concentrate and increase the capacity for learning and memory. Beginners are advised to start with the opening and closing actions of the palms, and practice the actions of the knees only after the feeling of qi has been experienced with certainty.

Patients with dizziness and headache are advised to practice the actions in the mind only moderately, concentrating instead on the physical actions. Practice of the opening and closing actions in the mind in the lying form before sleep is quite effective for treating insomnia and gastrointestinal conditions. In these cases, after a sufficient feeling of qi has appeared, the palms should be slowly dropped on the lower abdomen for concentration on Dantian (3 cun below the umbilicus)—that is, attention to the rise and fall as well as the feeling of opening and closing at Dantian.

Practice of the opening and closing actions of the knees is good for patients with cardiac palpitation. Consistent practice can also lower the blood pressure and relieve dizziness in those suffering from hypertension.

25

"Rocking on the Waves"
A Kind of Self-Massage

"Rocking on the waves" is a kind of self-massage exercise that, if properly practiced, is effective for gastrointestinal conditions such as constipation or diarrhea.

As the name implies, "rocking on the wave" is an exercise that makes the body swing to and fro like a wave. When doing the exercise, take a sitting position, and gently rotate and swing the upper torso to exercise the internal organs and the skeleton of the whole body so that the function of the channels and collaterals will be promoted, qi and blood circulation regulated and the internal organs strengthened.

"Rocking on the wave" is a simple exercise; even the weak, older people or invalids can practice it, provided that they are able to sit up.

Instructions

Sit as normal or with the legs crossed. Place the hands just proximal to the knees. Keeping the head upright and the spine straight, with the nose in line with the umbilicus, sit still and naturally for a while. Then relax the body and bend over from the right downwards, followed by turning to the left and raising the upper torso to form a full circle by returning to the original posture. Continue the movements without interruption. Rock to form 36 circles.

Repeat the action in the opposite direction, bending over from the left, turning to the right and raising the upper torso to form a full circle by returning to the original posture. Again, rock to form 36 circles.

This is a simple but effective exercise.

Notes

1. If a normal sitting position is taken, it is better to sit on a bench, not on the whole bench but only on its outer edge, about 10 cm into the bench. Keep the feet parallel and shoulder width apart. The key is not to splay the feet.

2. If a cross-legged sitting position is taken, rotate from the right to the left when the left leg is crossed on the right one, and rotate from the left to the right when the right leg is crossed on the left one. In other words, change the crossed leg when the direction of rotation is changed.

3. When the body is bent over and turning, take the waist as the axis and always keep the nose in line with the umbilicus. Don't raise the head.

4. The degree of bending over depends on the condition of the disease and the comfort level of the patient. Those suffering from hypertension with dizziness and those with a stuffy feeling in the chest should bend over to a lesser degree; those with soreness in the back and limbs, to a greater degree; and those with gastrointestinal diseases, to a moderate degree.

5. Slowness, evenness, relaxation and tranquility are required for the practice. While doing the exercise, imagine that you are floating in a sea of air and merging into a single whole with this sea of air.

"Rocking on the waves" can be used in both the treatment and prevention of disease. For therapeutic purposes, the number of rocking movements may be increased, but for preventive purposes it is sufficient to practice 36 circles each when turning to the left and to the right, taking about 15 minutes in total.

26

Health Exercise for the Prevention of Colds

According to the theory of meridians and collaterals in traditional Chinese medicine, acupuncture, moxibustion or massage on certain points may promote the circulation of qi and blood in the meridians and collaterals, which will mobilize the defensive power of the human body and increase the body's resistance to disease. Massage of the following acupoints may prevent and treat colds with fever and cough.

The exercise to prevent colds consists of four steps.

I. Rubbing the nose

Preparatory posture: Interlock the fingers of both hands and rub the fleshy part of the thumbs hot.

Movements: Interlock the fingers as before and rub the nose from the forehead downwards along the sides of the nose to Yingxiang (LI 20) (located in the nasolabial fold, 0.5 cun lateral to the alanasi) 16 times (see Fig. 1).

Functions: This promotes local circulation of qi and blood, resisting against the invasion of exogenous pathogens.

Requirements: Rub with moderate force.

II. Pressing Hegu (LI 4)

Movements: Press on the left Hegu (LI 4) (located on the dorsum of the hand, between the first and second metacarpal bones) with the right thumb and rotate the thumb to and fro for 16 turns. Then press the right Hegu (LI 4) with the left thumb and rotate it to and fro also for 16 turns (see Fig. 2).

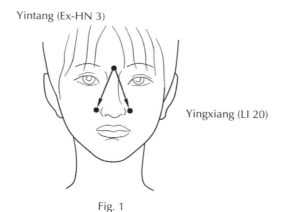

Yintang (Ex-HN 3)

Yingxiang (LI 20)

Fig. 1

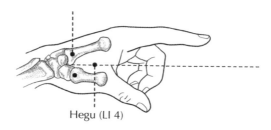

Hegu (LI 4)

Fig. 2

Functions: This has the function of removing pathogens from the surface of the body.

Requirements: The location of the acupoint should be accurate. (When the thumb and forefinger are spread, and the crease of the distal phalange of the opposite thumb is placed on the border of the web between the above-mentioned digits, Hegu (LI 4) is located at the tip of the opposite thumb.) Rub with appropriate force, inducing a sensation of soreness and distension.

III. Rubbing the face and pulling the ears

Preparatory posture: Rub the palms together until they feel hot.

Movements: Place the palms close to the forehead, moving downwards along the sides of the nose to the mandible while rubbing. Then move along the lateral sides of the face. When the hands pass the ears, gently pull the ear lobes outwards with the thumb and forefinger (see Fig. 3). Repeat 16 times.

Functions: Rubbing the face improves local blood circulation. The ear is the sea where the channels congregate, so pulling the ear lobe has the function of protecting health.

Requirements: The palms should maintain close contact with the face to produce a hot feeling during rubbing. After being pinched by the fingers and pulled outwards, the ear lobes are reddened.

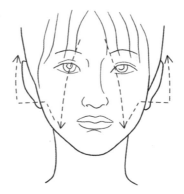

Fig. 3

IV. Kneading Yingxiang (LI 20)

Movements: Knead bilateral Yingxiang (LI 20) with the fingers.

Functions: Massage of this point promotes air flow through the nose.

Requirements: Locate the acupoint accurately and knead with appropriate force.

Note the following points when doing the exercise to prevent colds:

1. Clean the hands and cut the nails short before practice.

2. Perform the exercise once daily without interruption.

27

Protection of Health by "Hair-Combing"

Is there a relationship between maintenance of health and combing of hair? This had been studied in ancient China and the results were recorded in the literature. For example, *Qing Nong Lu* (Records of Getting Clean) points out: "Besides diet and Daoyin (physical and breathing exercises), there are two things crucial to the maintenance of health, i.e., combing of the hair and washing of the feet"; "Combing the hair and washing the feet benefit longevity and induce a peaceful sleep." *Zhu Bing Yuan Hou Lun* (General Treatise on the Causes and Symptoms of Diseases) advises: "Combing the hair for more than a thousand times will prevent the hair from getting gray." And *Yan Shou Shu* (On Prolonging the Life) states: "Frequent combing of the hair can improve vision and dispel wind."*

---

* "Wind" in traditional Chinese medicine refers to any disease or syndrome characterized by a sudden change of symptoms, such as stroke, which is manifested by the sudden onset of paralysis and impairment of consciousness.

Therefore, frequent combing of the hair not only nourishes the hair and dispels wind and fire,** but it also benefits general health. Of course, what was called "combing the hair" in ancient times did not really mean the use of a comb on the hair. It was a kind of massage on the head with hands instead of a comb. This method of health protection has been handed down from generation to generation through practice.

Instructions

Massage the head by scratching on the following seven acupoints:

1. Cuanzhu (B 2): in the depression at the head of the eyebrow.

2. Shenting (GV 24): on the anterior midline of the head, 0.5 cun superior to the anterior of the anterior hairline.

3. Qianding (GV 21): on the anterior midline of the head, 1.5 cun anterior to Baihui (GV 20), the midpoint of the line extending over the vertex joining the apexes of the auricles.

4. Naohu (GV 17): the key point for hair-combing, on the posterior midline of the head, in the depression superior to the upper border of the occipital protuberance.

** "Fire" in its traditional sense refers to pathological changes resulting from hyperactivity or emotional agitation with such manifestations as flushed face, bloodshot eyes, headache and irritability. Local inflammation is also considered a fire syndrome.

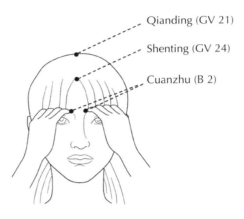

Qianding (GV 21)

Shenting (GV 24)

Cuanzhu (B 2)

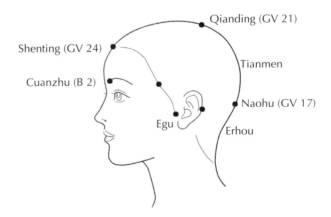

Qianding (GV 21)

Shenting (GV 24)

Tianmen

Cuanzhu (B 2)

Naohu (GV 17)

Egu

Erhou

5. Erhou: in the depression inferior to the mastoid process behind the ear.

6. Egu: immediately inferior to the ear.

7. Tianmen: the bony part immediately superior to the ear.

Actions

1. Bend the fingers into a rake. Place the tip of the thumb on Tianmen and the tip of the little finger on Cuanzhu (B 2), separating the remaining fingers with equal distance in between. Use both hands. This is the preparatory posture.

2. Move the hands upwards and backwards with force as if scratching an itch. Let the little finger pass through Shenting (GV 24) to Qianding (GV 21), and press Naohu (GV 17) with the forefingers. Then press bilateral Erhou with the thumbs and move the thumbs to Egu and then to Tianmen. The whole series of manipulation takes about 5 seconds. After the manipulation, the blood circulation of the skull will be activated.

Proper massage of these seven acupoints has a brain-tonifying action to prevent and treat dizziness and a feeling of distension in the head. Furthermore, consistent practice can promote the growth and restoration of the color to the hair, smooth the skin of the face and remove age spots. In some bald persons, new hair grows.

Notes

Perform the practice at an appropriate speed, not too fast nor too slow. Keep yourself in high spirits and practice consistently, "combing the hair" 30 times in the morning and in the evening for 1 to 2 minutes. Any posture can be taken while doing the practice: lying, sitting or standing.

28

Laozi's Brain-Tonifying Exercise

Laozi, one of the great thinkers of ancient China, was the founder of Taoism. Legend has it that he designed a series of exercises as a brain tonic that can be described as follows:

1. "Open" Yingtang (Ex-HN 3): Yingtang (Ex-HN 3) is in the midpoint between the eyebrows. First apply rotatory massage with the thumb tips to bilateral Taiyang (Ex-HN 5) and then knead Yingtang (Ex-HN 3) 16 times with the tips of the index fingers.

2. Rub the eyes: Rub both eyes around the orbits simultaneously 16 times with the tips of the index fingers.

3. "Push" Dicang (S 4): Dicang (S 4) is located 0.4 cun lateral to the corner of the mouth. Open the mouth a little. Press bilateral Dicang (S 4) with the tips of both thumbs, and push them up and down 16 times.

4. Press Sibai (S 2): Sibai (S 2) is located about 0.5 cun below the orbit. Press bilateral Sibai (S 2) with the tips of the index fingers obliquely from bottom to top 16 times.

5. Rub the nose: Rub the nose with the pads of the thumbs 16 times.

6. Rub the neck: Rub both sides of the neck with the palms 16 times.

7. Rub the face: Rub the face with the palms 16 times.

8. "Comb" the hair: Spread the fingers and rub the head with the fingertips somewhat forcefully from the forehead to the occiput, massaging the main channels on the head. "Comb" 16 times.

9. "Sound the heaven's drums": "Heaven's drum" refers to the ear. Cover the ears with the palms. Place the tip of the thumb on the middle finger and apply 16 flips on Fengchi (G 20) at the base of the skull below the occipital bone, which makes the sound "dong, dong."

After completing the nine steps, cover the ears tightly with the palms for a while and then remove the palms. Repeat three to five times. That is the end of the exercise.

29

Protection of the Teeth

In a fresco 4 meters high and 10 meters long found in Cave No. 196 of the Thousand-Buddha Grotto in Dunhuang, an old but healthy and strong-looking man who resembles a monk was painted. He is squatting on the ground, holding a bottle of water in his left hand and putting his right forefinger on his teeth—a vivid portrayal of teeth brushing. The fresco indicates that as early as 1,500 years ago people paid attention to teeth cleaning.

Among the unearthed relics, toothbrushes have been found that were made of animal bones from the Liao Dynasty more than 1,000 years ago. Dental caries was recorded as a common disease in the script on tortoise shells and animal bones 3,000 years ago.

In China's earliest medical classic—the Yellow Emperor's Canon of Medicine, written in the Warring States Period (475–221 BC)—the physiological phenomena of normal teeth were described. Since then, the Chinese have adopted measures for protecting teeth besides rinsing the mouth and brushing the teeth with toothpaste after meals and before sleep.

Teeth tapping is one of the measures.

Teeth tapping is the tapping of the upper and lower teeth on one another. More than 1,500 years ago, Ge Hong, a Jin Dynasty specialist in maintaining health, wrote in *Bao Pu Zi* (The Book of Master Baopu): "The teeth will never get loose if they are tapped for more than three hundred times every morning."

In China it has been found that many people who are in the habit of gritting their teeth during urination and defecation have a long life. Through gritting the teeth, massage is applied to their roots, promoting local blood circulation and nutrient supply, and thus strengthening the teeth. Since the digestive system starts from the teeth, having good teeth is certainly beneficial to health. Strong teeth and teeth tapping are the "secret" to longevity.

Instructions

Traditional teeth tapping is done in the following steps:

In the morning after getting up or in the evening before going to sleep, tap on the molars first, the incisors next and then the canines. They should be tapped separately because they are not on the same horizontal plane.

After the tapping, lick the gums and buccal mucosa with the tongue to stimulate secretion of saliva. Gargle with the saliva several times and then swallow it. In traditional Chinese medicine, saliva is considered a kind of body fluid that should not be expectorated.

Then massage the gums with the tongue, thereby improving blood circulation to the gums. Then grit the teeth and puff out the cheeks to increase salivary secretion. Swallow the saliva in several gulps.

This teeth-protection exercise can be done in about 10 minutes with 40 to 50 repetitions of the above-mentioned actions. Of course, the more repetitions you do, the better the results.

30

Exercise for the Hands and Feet

Traditional Chinese medicine holds that in the human body there are 12 meridians—three Yin meridians of the hand, three Yin meridians of the foot, three Yang meridians of the hand and three Yang meridians of the foot—that make up the main part of the meridians and collateral system in which nutrients, qi (vital energy) and blood circulate. This system plays an important role in both physiological functions and pathological changes.

The three Yin meridians of the hand run from the chest to the hands; the three Yang meridians of the hand run from the hands to the head; the three Yin meridians of the foot run from the feet to the abdomen; and the three Yang meridians of the foot run from the head to the feet. These are the main directions, though there are various other complicated courses.

Based on the theory of meridians and collaterals, exercising the hands and feet is particularly useful for regulating the functions of the heart and brain to prevent and treat cardiac and cerebral vascular diseases.

Instructions

Sit upright in a chair (don't lean on the chair back), keeping the back straight, chest pushed out, abdomen pulled in, shoulders relaxed, and upper arms hanging down naturally with a gap in each armpit as if holding an egg there. Bend the elbows and extend the forearms to the front of the chair with the palms facing down and fingers slightly bent. Touch the palate with the tongue, clench the molar teeth and gently shut the eyes (see Fig. 1).

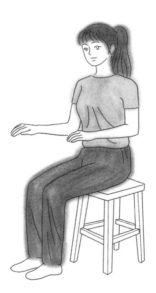

Fig. 1

Slowly bend the index finger inward to touch the palm as closely as possible and keep it in this position for 20 seconds to one minute. Then extend it slowly. Next move the ring finger in the same way, followed by the thumb, little finger and middle finger (see Figs 2, 3, 4, 5 and 6).

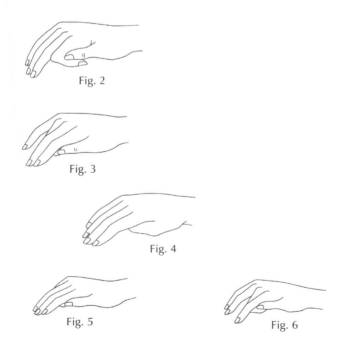

Fig. 2

Fig. 3

Fig. 4

Fig. 5

Fig. 6

It is better to move the corresponding toe when moving the finger. Moving a toe individually is difficult, but it can be tried with effort in the same order as the fingers. With practice, it will be possible to move individual toes.

After moving all the fingers, turn the palms up and gradually raise them, at the same time inhaling deeply through the nose. When the hands are raised above the chest, turning the hands down again, move them downward with pressure and exhale through the mouth (see Figs 7 and 8). After three to five repetitions, the exercise is concluded.

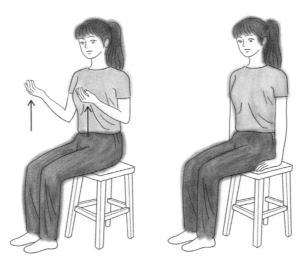

Fig. 7   Fig. 8

31

"Hungry Tiger Stretches Itself"
A Simple Health-Improving Exercise

"Hungry tiger stretches itself" is the name of an exercise in the famous Chinese martial art of Wudang. As a martial arts training move, it can greatly increase the ability to give a sudden blow. But if used as a therapeutic exercise, it has a remarkable effect on respiratory, cardiovascular and digestive diseases.

The exercise consists of a series of actions accomplished in a stretch. When it is repeated in cycles, it is sometimes full of power and grandeur, and sometimes mild and lingering. Thus, in the exercise hardness alternates with softness, rapidity with slowness, and both the functions of the internal organs and physical strength are invigorated. It is in fact a combination of static and dynamic exercises.

Preparatory posture: Stand with the feet parallel and a little more than shoulder width apart.

Key points: Keep the head upright, eyes looking forward, chin tucked in, face natural, shoulders and chest relaxed, arms hanging down by the sides of the body, fingers somewhat separated, palm centers hollowed, buttocks pulled in, anus constricted, legs slightly bent with knees close to each other, soles and toes touching the ground with the sole centers hollowed, and imagining that the soles are sinking into the ground like the roots of a big tree.

Think about and concentrate on each part of the body in the order mentioned above, repeating this mental examination three times to discharge the turbid qi throughout the body together with the flow of thought. The preparatory form itself is a kind of static exercise for health protection and can be practiced alone.

The actions of "hungry tiger stretching itself" are as follows:

1. "Blowing wind into the ears": Move the arms from the sides of the body upwards and outwards to form two arcs, the palms facing down. Meanwhile, the flow of thought goes down from the waist and hips through the knees to the soles, accompanied by slow and smooth inhalation. When the palms reach shoulder level, inwardly rotate the forearms and slightly bend the elbows, with the backs of the hands facing each other, the thumbs pointing down and the fingers pointing to the front, as if the wind were blowing into both ears.

Continuing the action and inhalation, turn the hands to make the palms face forward and place that part of the hand between thumb and forefinger at eye level, arching the arms as shown in Fig. 1.

2. "Tiger sitting on a mountaintop": Immediately after the preceeding action, start exhaling slowly and smoothly. Move the hands back to either side of the ears and curl the fingers as if holding a ball, so that the palms look like tiger's claws. Dropping the shoulders and elbows and pushing out the chest, direct qi down to Dantian, the area 3.0 cun below the umbilicus (see Fig. 2).

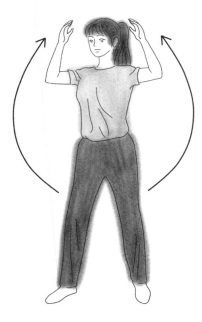

Fig. 1

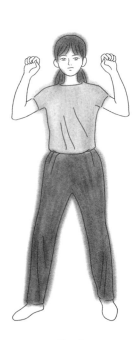

Fig. 2

3. "Stretching out the tiger's claws": Inhaling slowly and smoothly, stretch the "tiger's claws" forwards, wrists bending backwards, palms facing front, forearms twisting inwards, cubital fossae facing upwards, and elbows dropped. Relax the chest, pull in the abdomen and buttocks and straighten the lumbar spine, eyes looking at the hands (see Fig. 3).

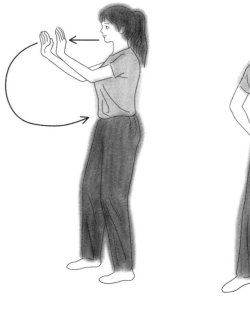
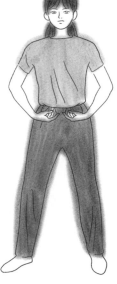

Fig. 3   Fig. 4

4. "Hungry tiger pouncing on its prey": While taking a deep breath, turn the "tiger's claws" downwards, then inwards (palms facing the lower abdomen) and finally upwards (palms facing up). Arch the arms as shown in Fig. 4. Hold the breath to accumulate strength, and then breathe out a little.

5. "Pushing the mountain with force": Rapidly and forcefully rotate the forearms inwards, turning the palms to face front. Dropping the shoulders and elbows, and bending the wrists backwards, push the palms forwards at the height of the shoulders, with qi penetrating into the roots of the palms and fingertips. Meanwhile, bend the knees and squat down to form a horseman's stance, exhaling air in a burst of sound ("hei"), with the lumbar spine pushed out and the anus constricted, as shown in Fig. 5.

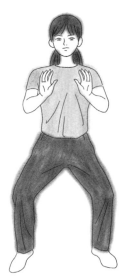

Fig. 5

Note: In martial training, this action is violent and rapid. However, for the purpose of a therapeutic exercise, it should be gentle and slow, accompanied by the flow of thought but not by force.

6. "Tiger's play in the mountain": Slowly exhaling the remaining air, turn the "tiger's claws" into palms extending straight forward, with qi penetrating from the roots of the palms into the fingertips. Rotate the forearms outwards, and turn the palms outwards in two arcs with the thumbs leading from the medial to the lateral and the palms from facing front to facing down and finally to facing up. Retract, bend and lower the arms, gradually moving the elbows outwards with the fingers of both hands pointed towards one another. At the same time, rise up slowly and smoothly to an upright position and start inhaling (see Fig. 6).

After this action, return to the first action ("Blowing wind into the ears"). The six actions, forming one cycle, should be performed in succession without interruption and accompanied by two respirations. At each practice 9 to 36 cycles are necessary. The exercise is characterized by the rising and falling of the limbs, continuation of action, natural and even breathing, and smooth and agile movement.

Concluding form: After the sixth action of the last cycle, return to the posture in the first action. Turn the palms from facing front to facing down, and then slowly move the hands downwards accompanied by smooth exhalation until the hands reach the front of the lower abdomen. Along with the movement of the arms, the internal qi also descends from Baihui (CV 20) on the vertex of the head down to Dantian in the abdomen. Lower the arms further and return to the preparatory form. Finally, breathe nine times to conclude the exercise.

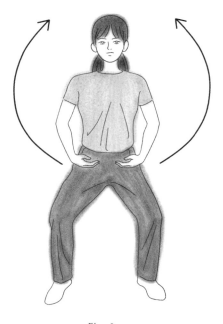

Fig. 6